Head Lights

for

Dark Roads:

Packing Humor and Hope
for the Unexpected Trip
through Traumatic Brain Injury

Diane Quimby

Vabella Publishing
P.O. Box 1052
Carrollton, Georgia 30112
www.vabella.com

©Copyright 2012 by Diane Quimby

Cover art by Jesse Duke
Cover design by Brady Parks

Manufactured in the United States of America

13-digit ISBN 978-1-938230-13-4

Library of Congress Control Number 2012944855

10 9 8 7 6 5 4 3 2 1

For Andy Lane, who sustained a spinal cord injury in 1981, and taught me how to face catastrophic injury with courage and humor. And for all survivors of traumatic brain injury and for their caregivers who face their own courageous journeys. May you never lose hope, and in the face of all challenges…Endure!

Traumatic Brain Injury Conference

The smiley face sticker on my nametag
warns everyone around me.
She is not like us.
She is one of them.

A conference of professionals
making mortgage payments
on my dime.
They are the experts.

When did I become diminished?
Was it the impact of head and airbag?
Or when I woke from the coma?
Or the moment I put on the smiley face?

Finally, she sits by me at lunch and asks,
"Did they tell you that you wouldn't
improve after a year?"
She sees the answer in my eyes.

"Don't listen to them," she says.
"That is bullshit!"
Years later, and I still think
of that shining moment.

She popped a cherry tomato into
her mouth as if nothing had happened.
Yet, years later, I still remember
the moment I found hope.

Diane Quimby
2008

Foreword

In many ways the Shepherd family has been my inspiration. In 1973, Harold and Alana Shepherd learned that their son James had received a paralyzing injury while body surfing in Brazil. There was no specialized facility in the Southeast that could meet his needs. Their son James had to travel to Denver to receive treatment.

Working within the Atlanta Community, these three remarkable people have been the catalyst and driving force in establishing one of the finest rehabilitation and treatment facilities in the country for spinal cord injury and acquired brain injury. I count myself among the thousands of people who are living independent and full lives today because of their vision and desire to help others. I am following their example when I donate all profits from the sale of this book to traumatic brain injury organizations.

These stories about my peers provide a voice and honor the incredible people who have shared this journey of pain and joy with me during our darkest days. Although some may no longer remember clearly enough to share these lessons I have been witness to, their remarkable lives have changed me forever. I honor them for what they have taught me. Their courage was a light for me in the darkness until I found courage for myself. I hope their extraordinary spirit shines through on the page. All names of patients and caregivers have been excluded or changed to protect their privacy.

The spiritual lessons learned on my continuing journey through traumatic brain injury are written to encourage those behind me. I hope I have exposed common pitfalls, and have offered encouragement and hope for both the survivor and the caregiver.

For my family who will read this, I want to thank you. As soon as the tracheotomy tube was removed and I could speak, I announced that I was going to write a book. I don't remember saying this, but when I was reminded of it later the seed was planted. As I became more aware, I began to make notes of other patients and my experiences. Without those notes many of these memories would have been lost, and I could not have written this book. Without your encouragement and love I could not have stuck with it. I hope that you will not be disappointed.

Finally, every brain injury is unique. This book is my personal journey. However, all TBI survivors and caregivers share many of the same roads, and I hope that I have left clear markers to make the journey easier.

I know that God will keep you close. I pray that you will keep God close.

Above all else – Endure!

Diane

Endurance is not just the ability to bear a hard thing, but to turn it into glory. ~ William Barclay

*Every Step in the dark turns out in the end
to have been on course after all.*

~John Tarrant

First Thoughts

Sound could not penetrate this heavy curtain of darkness. Chilly, but strangely humid, this darkness was deeper than black and so heavy that I could feel its dampness touching the hairs on my arms. My eyes were wide open, yet I could not see. I didn't need to. I knew exactly where I was. I stood on a high precipice. Just one step forward and all would be over. I felt no fear, but I did not move. I was waiting . . .

No voice, no sound, but a thought like the loud clap of thunder shouted, and I felt the presence of luminous warmth behind me. Slowly and deliberately without turning I stepped back from the abyss – toward the presence I knew was God.

These were my first thoughts.

Stillness in stillness is not the real stillness. Only when there is stillness in movement can the spiritual rhythm appear which pervades heaven and earth.

~Taoist Saying

First Words

I was suddenly aware that someone was close to me speaking in my ear. The voice said, "My name is Scott Quimby. I am your husband. We have been married for twenty-eight years and I love you with all of my heart." He hugged me and moved back so that I could see him. I looked intently at him. He had kind eyes, but I did not recognize the man. Then, gradually as I continued to stare at him, I understood that he was Scott, and I remembered! These first words are seared into my memory and that is a miracle, because this was my first conscious thought in over a month and my only distinct memory of my six-week stay at Memorial University Medical Center in Savannah, GA.

I didn't know that I had just come out of a coma. I didn't know that I was seeing him for the first time in over a month. I didn't know that it would soon be Christmas. I didn't remember the car accident on November third, and I didn't realize that I had a tracheotomy tube in my throat and could not speak. I knew just one thing. Scott was here and that was enough.

Miracles are a retelling in small letters of the very same story, which is written across the whole world in letters too large for some of us to see. ~ C.S. Lewis

New Eyes

It seems ironic that I would awaken in a hospital named *Memorial* University Medical Center and have so few memories of my six-week stay. I have some memory of the last few days I was there, but they are blurred flashes in a broken perspective. I vaguely remember being frustrated and writing something to my brother Doug. Much later he explained that he came to visit me and found me extremely agitated. Since I could not yet speak, he tried to get me to write down what was wrong. I tried many times to write, but each time it looked like scribble. I was finally able to write a sentence he could read. As he explained this to me, he pulled a folded paper out of his wallet that he had saved from months before. It was filled with scribbles and a single sentence that was barely legible. The message said, "I want justice."

After the tracheotomy tube was removed and I could speak, my family learned what I was thinking, and uneasiness swept over them. I made no sense. It was my brother Doug who seemed to have the hardest time dealing with my lack of cognitive ability. He put me through a battery of questions at each visit. Although I don't remember our specific conversation, he reminded me of it much later when I could think and remember. It went something like this:

"Diane, do you know where you are?"

3

"Yes," I told him confidently, "I am in the hospital." He breathed a sigh of relief, and if he had let the questioning end there he would have felt much better in thinking that I was improving.

"Exactly where is the hospital located? Where are you?"

I must have wondered what was wrong with him. Didn't he know where we were? "I'm in Mexico."

"What? Mexico? Why are you in Mexico?"

"I got shot."

"Shot?" he repeated in an increasingly concerned voice. "Why were you shot?"

"In the war!" I shouted. I don't remember this conversation, but I do remember feeling very frustrated that he didn't know about the war.

My husband Scott and a good friend, also named Diane, had an equally weird conversation with me about one of the nurses. She was from England, and I was certain that she was a British spy. When she came into the room I strictly forbade anyone from talking to her. If they did, I became very upset. I was convinced that she was sending any information gathered while in my room to our adversaries in the war. Later, as I was prepared for transfer to Shepherd Center in Atlanta, I was lying on a stretcher and I remember that she bent down and kissed me on the cheek. I physically could not prevent her from doing this, and it distressed me deeply. Now I am equally disturbed that I didn't thank her for her patience and care.

Poor Doug. It seemed that I was always most bizarre with him. I think it is because he questioned me more, trying to understand what was impossible to understand. How can anyone understand the inner workings of an injured brain? Scott didn't question. He just accepted it all, and quietly kept faith that the person he had known for so long would fight her way out of this jumbled world of confusion to find reason, and ultimately regain a sense of self.

Later, Doug reminded me of another conversation. The doctor had just left my room when Doug arrived, and I told him that I had sustained approximately 61 fractures in the car wreck.

He looked at me with a puzzled expression and said, "You told me 76 fractures last night. Where did the number 76 come from?"

In all sincerity, and with no sense at how strange this would sound, I started singing the first two lines of a show tune from the Broadway musical, *The Music Man*. "Seventy-six trombones led the big parade. With a hundred and ten cornets close at hand..." I don't remember this impromptu aria, but I'm sure that he laughed, and then began to worry even more.

In between these moments of chaotic thought I had vivid hallucinations. I still remember two quite distinctly. One I will detail in a later story, and one was quite a nightmare about a hideous alien who got on a ferry with me.

Although they visited frequently, I still have no memory of seeing my mom and dad, my children, or any other close friend or family member not already mentioned.

And frankly, I didn't miss them. I was experiencing too much data for my brain to process. I was in a constant state of being that alternated between overload and complete meltdown. Occasionally I would have an experience that I can still remember, although I cannot put the memory into any context. The only exception is the very lucid and distinct memory of when I first heard and saw Scott. I will always consider this memory my greatest gift of comfort and reassurance from God, and I continue to cherish this memory. I considered the experiences I did not remember as insignificant since these experiences failed to connect and become long-term memory. However, a conversation with my mom two years later changed my mind. I was visiting her in Tennessee. She and I were talking over morning coffee. We began to reminisce about my accident. I asked her if she had worried that I would never improve from the brain injury.

She looked at me for a long moment and asked, "You don't remember when I sat with you that afternoon in Savannah, do you?"

"No, mom I don't remember seeing you there at all."

She was quiet for a few moments. Her eyes filled with tears as she spoke. "You were asleep when I came into your room. When you woke, you looked around, and when you saw me, you said, 'There's an angel sitting in the chair beside you, Mom. Can you see him?'"

She had answered, "No, I can't see him." She told me that I calmly looked at the other chair and described him in great detail. He was dark skinned, with dark eyes, and dark hair. His clothes were light in color and seemed to somehow be illuminated from inside.

She confided that when she left my room that day, she knew that I was going to get better. At this time I was still unable to think coherently, unable to sit up, unable to walk, unable to feed or dress myself. She shared that if she had assessed my situation using her eyes, she would have questioned my ability to ever have an independent or fulfilling life. She made a decision to rely on the assessment of my situation using my eyes, and she left convinced that I would find a way back.

The real voyage of discovery consists not in seeking new landscapes, but in having new eyes.
~ Marcel Proust

Going to Mars

Scott came into my room and told me that I would be leaving Savannah to go to Shepherd Center in Atlanta and that he would be with me in the ambulance as I traveled there. I understood that I would leave, and that he would be with me, but the rest was too much to understand. He seemed so excited, so I gave him a smile and remembered nothing else that was said.

He could have been saying, "Diane, tomorrow we are loading you on a spaceship for Mars!" and I would have reacted the same. It was only his enthusiasm that told me wherever I was going was a good place. The trip to Atlanta was hazy and nondescript with one exception. While being transferred from the ambulance into the hospital, the mid-December wind gently blew an unseasonably warm breeze. It had been six weeks since I had felt the wind on my face. I felt such joy at the sensation. It felt glorious!

I remember nothing else of my arrival at Shepherd. Much later I would learn that I fired everyone I saw, and I took a swing at a therapist named Therese. Even today, when I visit the ABI (Acquired Brain Injury) unit at Shepherd Center volunteering as a peer visitor, I will invariably come across someone who tells me that I fired them. My six-week stay in Savannah was behind me; having been in a coma for the first month and heavily sedated and confused the other two weeks, I remember almost nothing of my stay. However, nothing that happened in Savannah prepared me for what I would face at Shepherd Center.

After a brief evaluation period I was introduced to the Shepherd schedule that I still refer to as boot camp. Life in the ABI unit could have easily been the planet Mars, because everything I experienced there was foreign to me except for the early start each morning. As I was weaned off of the heavy doses of pain medications I began to understand what had happened to me. This understanding took weeks and I am thankful for that. There are some things you must learn gradually. I don't believe the human mind, especially an injured one, can assimilate massive injury and loss all at once. To know the extent of all of my injuries would have broken my spirit.

I remember the first morning I awoke on a lower dose of pain medication. I felt an ache of pain and looked over at my right hand. It was lying at a 45-degree angle from my wrist. I remember thinking *this can't be good*. Both of my feet and legs were in casts. I began to take an inventory on this new body that I was housed in.

There was a long vertical scar that ran from beneath my breast area to a few inches below my navel (or what had once been a navel). Another scar ran horizontal. There were scars of holes where life-saving equipment had been installed and taken out. Both of my hands and left arm had numerous scars. I had no sensation of feeling in my right leg and both feet, and in various parts of my body. There was a colostomy bag attached on my left side. Yes, this body definitely could have, and should have belonged to someone living on Mars.

Weeks later I saw my image in a mirror. The left side of my face was frozen in paralysis and when I tried to smile it looked like I was snarling. My left eye would not close and was widely open, requiring medication to keep it lubricated. I even looked like an alien from Mars.

Each morning I was cleaned, and was hoisted up in a machine that looked like a miniature crane and placed in a wheelchair. Unable to fully use my arms I was pushed to a common waiting area to await the arrival of breakfast. From 9:00 until 3:00 every day, with a break for lunch, I was pushed to my physical and mental limits. This physical therapy was grueling hard work. It was harder than anything I have ever experienced.

The constant pain of being in a wheelchair with three fractures in my pelvis, a fractured tailbone, two fractured vertebrae, and fractured ribs still mending only complicated the whole ordeal. The therapists at Shepherd were absolutely amazing. In six short weeks I went from being unable to sit unassisted outside of my chair to actually standing and walking a few steps with the aid of an apparatus that looked like a wheeled, padded crucifix with arm rests. Even the equipment looked Martian made.

These six weeks at Shepherd were the hardest and most important six weeks in my life. There are no words to explain the pain and joy, the frustration and triumph, the moments of simple victories that I experienced. I learned to manipulate various devices to help me as I relearned how to bathe, how to dress, how to put on socks and shoes, and how to brush my teeth. The device I learned to use to put on socks looked weird, but it worked. These Martians had thought of everything.

The teacher who taught me to master all of these devices and basic functions was Therese, the woman I had taken a swing at when I was first admitted. She never told me this. I learned it much later. For every act of independence I now perform, she is responsible.

There are days when I awake spiritually sharp. On these days I sit up, swing my legs over the bed, and *walk* into the bathroom. I shower, brush my teeth, and dress, and with each function I perform, I invariably think of Therese. I thank God for her life. She was one of my greatest guides while visiting the planet Mars.

It's very hard to take yourself too seriously when you look at the world from outer space.
~ Astronaut Thomas K. Mattingly II

Bingo Prayers

It was my first day in a therapy class called Life Skills, and the bingo game had just begun. The recreational therapist retrieved a bingo ball from the hand-cranked hopper.

"I-22," she called.

"What did she say?"

The therapist repeated the number, and Janice, a patient sitting next to me, pointed and said, "It's right there on your card."

"Where?" The game was temporarily halted while patients on each side of me helped me place my bingo marker on my card.

The therapist next called out "B-6".

"What did she say?" I asked again.

This time my question was answered by the stony stares of the other patients. The therapist, noticing tenseness in the silence, glanced up and quickly read the situation. I was in the ABI unit, and tempers here could flare. She quickly helped me place my bingo marker on the correct square.

Once again, after retrieving a bingo ball from the hopper she announced, "G-47." I still could not hear her, but one quick glance around the room convinced me not to interrupt the game. I had a brain injury, but I wasn't stupid. I decided to sit the game out.

For someone used to being in the middle of the action, sitting on the sidelines, unable to compete was hard to take. I began to feel the frustration I would experience many times in the recovery process. I began to feel sorry for myself. *I can't even play bingo.* I was disgusted with myself. For the first time in my life, I felt useless.

I glanced at the other patients as they concentrated on their bingo cards. A quick thought, completely contrary to my self-pitying mood came into my mind. *Pray for them.* What? *Pray for them* the thought nudged me again. I looked around at the other patients, and then silently and tentatively I began to pray for each person in the room.

As I prayed, the most amazing thing happened. I began to notice small details that I hadn't seen before. I saw the dark blue fingernail polish Cheryl wore. She appeared much younger than my first impression of her. Most of her hair had fallen out. She had short thin dark brown hair in random spots on her head. Her hair loss gave her the look of a much older woman. Being in a wheelchair and having limited arm movement must be even harder for someone in her early twenties. I would try to remember to compliment her later on her beautiful fingernails.

Janice, a teenager, had fewer physical ailments, but her brain injury was a great challenge. She could just keep up with the bingo game if she devoted all of her attention to the task. Her brow was knitted together in total concentration. She had the anger issues sometimes common with a head injury. I could tell she did not like the interruptions I was causing. I found myself praying that she would win the game. Win or lose, I promised myself, I would sit beside Janice at lunch and tell her what a great bingo player she was.

So it went with each person. I had been given a deeper perspective. I felt a keen awareness for each person as I prayed. Ideas to encourage others began to fill my mind. At the end of the hour I felt energized and I no longer felt useless. In fact, I felt excited! I decided to pray for the people that I met each day and look for ways to offer encouragement. Most important, I believed that God would answer my prayers.

I didn't realize it at the time, but this decision to pray for others taught me spiritual lessons about giving and receiving, the power of prayer, and the power of a focused mind. It is impossible to give so much of yourself without God filling you back up. As I continued to pray for others and offer them encouragement, they began to encourage each other and me. The physical therapy gym became even more positive than usual. What had once been a place of pain and fear of further injury was becoming a place of hope and small daily victories. Physically and mentally, I was still challenged, but spiritually I began to soar! Prayer and the change in my attitude had made all the difference.

I saw continual improvement in my new friends, and it excited me to realize that I was improving also. I could now sit up and maintain my balance. I was learning to wheel myself around in my wheelchair. That feat alone gave me greater mobility. In every place I looked, I saw improvement and answered prayers. I realized that prayer not only heals the person being prayed for, it also heals the person doing the praying!

Much later, after being diagnosed with severe hearing loss, I received new hearing aids and brand new prescription glasses. Once again, the bingo game was in full swing. Although I held my bingo card in my hand confident that I could finally play along I never bothered to cover a square. I remained focused on my mission.

I was busy praying for all of us when I heard someone yell, "Bingo!" Amid the inevitable groans of the losers, I looked up and smiled. Janice had finally won.

Another answered prayer!

None of us will ever accomplish
anything excellent or commanding
except when he listens to this whisper
which is heard by him alone.
~ Ralph Waldo Emerson

Night

Night was hardest to endure. There were the sounds of pain – sometimes moans, occasionally a yell – as someone had reached his or her limit and needed to vent. These were the sounds of my new home. These sounds and smells were a sterile and sometimes eerie environment. There was also the constant throbbing of pain and the cacophony of fears swirling in my head. Knowing that all too soon I would face a new day of therapy, and that I needed to rest for the energy to face a new day of challenges, made sleep as elusive as chasing a butterfly.

Time was an enemy that made night seem endless. It magnified the constant and unrelenting pain of wounds, and bones that ached as they knitted back together. Yes, the nights were definitely the worst. But in this time of despair, God's presence becomes stronger and more dynamic. It is in the night when all pretense of self is laid bare like an old chair that is being refinished. Each layer of paint and stain is removed, until at last, the original beauty of the wood is visible and the elegance and simplicity of the chair is revealed. That is how God revealed himself to me.

That is when God became my refuge and strength in time of trouble. All of the layers of vanity, ego, pride, and self-importance were stripped away. And like the chair, seeking God was gloriously revealed in the simplicity of a child who seeks a parent for comfort. There was no bargaining with God for health, no recriminations or what ifs, no bitterness, or ulterior motives; only to seek him for comfort and find peace in the dark recesses of my mind, and reassurance in my heart that I could conquer this – whatever this was, or would become. I could hang on and get through it. Until at last there was steel resolve, more impenetrable than any blast proof door that closes and locks out doubt.

During the night, I learned to recognize God for who he really is – *Love*. I began to understand his great love for me. I talked with him and confided my deepest fears, and I released them to him to carry for me. Some mornings I awoke to promptly take these burdens back and tried to carry them. But on the mornings that I left my fear with God, I accomplished great, small victories in my therapy.

As I sought God, I began to recognize his voice. It came as a still, small voice that was disguised as a thought. Yet, this thought was not according to how I felt, or what I would normally think. It was always simple, positive, and if I acted on these thoughts – powerful. It is easy to understand how the Apostle Paul sometimes doubted these thoughts were God – they are so very simple. Yet, in this simplicity, is the infinite power of the universe.

Faith is not making religious-sounding noises in the daytime. It is asking your inmost self questions at night – and then getting up and going to work.
~ Mary Jean Irion

Houdini

The three patients who shared a four-bed ward with him nicknamed him Houdini. He was eighteen years old and had been injured in a car accident. Although the doctors had determined that he was physically able to speak, he had not spoken since his wreck. Yet, without uttering one single word he possessed the most vibrant personality of all the patients I met at Shepherd Center. He kept the staff on their toes, and his resourcefulness and persistence were a constant source of amusement and entertainment for the other patients. In many ways he looked like a typical teenager, with short brown hair and an average build. A casual observer would notice this and no more.

However, a closer inspection would reveal two startling features: his eyes. He conveyed a complete lack of emotion in them. If the eyes are the windows to the soul, Jeremy's eyes had the shades drawn tight. There was no hint as to what he was thinking, no flicker of amusement or annoyance, only the collection of data and constant observation. His eyes scrutinized every patient, every therapist, every nurse, and every visitor. No person, no event was missed. Like a living, breathing camcorder, he recorded it all.

Although he could walk, he had balance problems which required temporary use of a wheelchair. This ensured that he didn't take any tumbles and receive further brain injury. He hated being in a wheelchair and spent considerable effort to escape the wheelchair and the ABI ward. He had developed quite a talent for escape. At first he was restrained with his wheelchair seat belt. Quickly a locked belt was added for safety.

With patience and practice he became quite skilled in picking the lock.

It was common to see him wandering the halls or hovering by the electronic door seeking an opportunity to bolt outside, and breathe in a few precious moments of freedom, before being rounded up and returned to the confines of the ABI ward.

He became an even greater menace during the night. He could escape any security measures the staff employed. His roommates often kept us in stitches during breakfast relaying Houdini's latest exploits of the night before. He was especially fond of raiding the staff refrigerator and eating their food. There was no doubt about it – he was going down as a legend in the ABI unit.

One morning at breakfast he sat directly across from me. Jeremy ate his breakfast quickly, and began to stare intently at my tray. He placed his hand on the table and began to run his hand slowly and deliberately toward my food. I watched, fascinated, wondering what he would do when his hand reached my tray. Just as his hand finally reached the edge of my tray, a tech noticed him and called his name. He slid his hand back and rolled away in his wheelchair.

The following week he was transferred to Pathways as a full time outpatient. He would be living at home and would come in each day for therapy. Over the next few weeks, I often wondered how he felt about his newfound freedom. Four weeks later, I was transferred as an inpatient to Pathways, and learned the answer.

On my first day as an inpatient at Pathways, I saw him. He walked into the lunchroom with two other guys his age. He smiled at something one of them said. I could not believe the change in his face. It was amazing to realize how a simple smile had completely transformed his appearance. His eyes, once dead, now had a twinkle of mischievousness and humor. I had only begun to take in this metamorphosis when the most miraculous thing happened. He looked at his friends and *spoke*. I watched in awe as he and his friends found a table together and began to eat their lunch. He looked like any other teenage boy sitting with his friends and talking. After lunch, the three friends went into the billiard room and shot a game of pool.

Over the next couple of weeks I kept a lookout for Jeremy. Outpatients brought their lunches in coolers. Jeremy's cooler reminded me of a cooler that Jethro Bodine, from *The Beverly Hillbillies,* might carry. It was huge and his mom packed it full every day. He always ate every bite. I was an inpatient. My perishable food was stored in the refrigerator or freezer. All inpatients were scheduled a weekly trip to the grocery store. I started buying Klondike ice cream bars. After his lunch each day, I would offer him an ice cream. He must have wondered at this woman who always gave him food. He was the same age as my oldest son, Anthony, and as I thought of this, I decided to care for him, as I would have liked someone to care for Anthony.

As we all left the lunchroom on that first day, I took the opportunity to speak to him. "Hi, Jeremy, it's good to see you again. Do you like it here?"

"Yeah, it's a lot better. They say I'm doing real good."

And he was. Three weeks later he was released to go home. Houdini had vanished, and in his place was a handsome, soft-spoken teenaged boy with a shy smile. I miss them both.

The most profound statements are often said in silence.
~ Lynn Johnston

Dead Batteries

When I think of the situation my husband found himself in, I don't know how he handled it all. One day everything was great. The next day he did not know if his wife would live. Once he knew that I would live, he found himself married to a woman locked up in a brain injury ward with no firm answers on how her brain might work in the future.

Years later he told me that he did not worry about the physical issues. He knew that we would work through them, but he could not find anyone who would guarantee how much I would improve from the brain injury. He confided that the biggest worry came from not knowing what to expect. Almost two weeks after I transferred to Shepherd, Scott got his answer in a way he never imagined.

Our daughter Kelly had brought me a CD player with headphones. She had burned a CD of songs from her play-list that she knew I would like. I wore these headphones all night, with the songs set to replay. My first roommate, Christina, was prone to be noisy at night and the headphones gave me an uninterrupted sleep. However, playing the CD player all night meant that I was using up AA batteries every couple of days. I had just come back from therapy and was resting in the bed when my batteries ran down. I really needed batteries for my CD player – I understood that much.

I don't remember how long I lay there considering this problem. How could I get batteries? I thought of Scott. He was coming to see me that night. If only he knew that I needed batteries. I lay in the bed and considered this problem. I noticed the telephone in the room. *Could I call Scott?* I began to feel overwhelmed and frustrated. Finally, I closed my eyes and thought hard. If I could just reach the phone sitting on the dresser near my bed, I could call Scott. I leaned over as far as I could and grabbed the phone.

The phone now sat on my lap. I picked it up, and then realized I could not remember Scott's phone number. I placed the receiver down and moved it off of my lap. I decided to take a nap. I closed my eyes and relaxed, and then a phone number came into my head as clear as a bell. I grabbed the phone and dialed it fast before the number was gone. As the phone began to ring I started to question that this was really Scott's number. *Suppose someone else answered? What would I say?* Fortunately, Scott answered on the second ring, because I was working myself into a panic attack over the possibility of dialing a wrong number.

"Hello," he said. I was thrilled to recognize his voice.

"Scott, this is Diane. Can you bring me some AA batteries when you come to see me tonight?" There was a long pause and I asked, "Scott, are you there?"

Finally, his voice said, "Yes, I am here." There was another long pause and then he asked, "Diane, how did you call me?"

"On the telephone."

"Yes, I know we are talking on the phone, but how did you call? Is someone there who helped you call me?"

22

"No," I told him, not understanding why he was questioning me. "I knew I needed batteries and I got the phone and called you."

There was another long pause, "How did you get my number?"

"I remembered it."

We talked briefly and then hung up. I was completely exhausted by the mental energy it had taken for me to make this phone call. I went to sleep.

At the time I did not understand the significance of performing this simple act. For someone who hadn't made any sense for almost two months, who couldn't remember or perform the most basic functions unassisted, this first step was huge! Scott told me much later that after we hung up he had been stunned, and had actually turned the telephone toward his face to stare at it.

His friends at work had been very supportive of him since my wreck. One of his friends saw him staring at his cell phone.

He anxiously asked, "Is everything okay?"

Scott looked at his friend with a smile of great relief on his face, and for the first time in two months that seemed a lifetime he said, "Yes, everything is fine. Everything really is going to be just fine."

A journey of a thousand miles begins with a single step.
~ Confucius

Roommate Roulette

Christina was an entertaining first roommate. Although she was in her thirties, she had the antics of a precocious twelve year old. Her bed looked like one of those canvas tents that store multicolored balls children play in. Her bed did not have the balls inside, but it did have a zippered screen to keep her in bed and out of mischief during the night.

Exuberant like a puppy that runs for the love of running, she was playful, happy, and easy to share a room with during the day. However, she was loud – especially at night. I learned to sleep with headphones on. Some nights, when I felt that I was only hanging on by a thread, I would set the CD player to repeat and listen to one song over and over...*Try, Try, Try* by the Smashing Pumpkins. The chorus contained the words *"Try to hold on."* That became my nighttime mantra.

Stevie arrived next. She was only there for a couple of days. She was a former Shepherd patient who had been re-admitted for a specific rehabilitation treatment and just as quickly she was gone. She was a lovely young woman with a fabulous husband. He was so kind to her, and I saw, in those few days, a marriage that looked as strong as one could ever hope for. It wasn't hard for me to imagine them aging into a remarkable couple with many experiences well beyond the confines of the ABI unit. I received a copy of *The*

Spinal Column, a quarterly Shepherd magazine, a year or so later. Under the heading of Alumni News, I was thrilled to see a beautiful photograph of her. The paragraph under her picture told of her successful re-entry into her old job, and her joy in her new life.

Donita became my third roommate. She came to Shepherd Center after me, but was transferred to Shepherd Pathways before me. She was a delightful person, and I really missed her. Later, when I was transferred to Pathways, we even performed a song together. She was a wonderful artist, and sketched pictures of her life at Shepherd. They revealed poignant moments, captured as no artist could have drawn without living through this ordeal. One of her sketches hung on the wall at Shepherd Pathways.

Rhoda was my final roommate. She was the most negative person I have ever encountered. She received her brain injury at the hands of an abusive boyfriend. She talked on the phone constantly. When talking to her friends she ranted about him while looking for ways to make him pay for all that he had done to her. Later, I could hear her talking to him in a hushed voice. I had no doubt that she had every intention of returning to this nightmare life upon her release.

I had visitors on her first night at Shepherd. We talked and laughed, and she could not stand the sounds of our laughter. I ended up being loaded back into my wheelchair and we concluded our visit in the patients' lounge. That first night was an omen of all that would come. My last week at Shepherd became a silent battle of wills – positive vs. negative, Luke Skywalker vs. The Emperor.

Negativity was her way of life. I often wondered what had happened to her in the past that condemned her to dream so small for her life. This life of abuse seemed so normal to her, and her negativity was so deep, that I felt sure she had never lived in a positive environment.

In the evenings, after my husband left, I got my CD player that had been stashed away since Christina left, back out of the drawer, and began to drown out my new roommate. Christina had been innocently loud, but Rhoda used words that wounded, and dragged down my spirit. With great relief, I soon left Shepherd and was transferred to Pathways.

In my year of therapy, and now as a volunteer, I have seen people horrendously broken. Some may never think at a level that will offer them any independence. I have seen people unable to communicate, and others who fought determinedly for every basic skill or function they could relearn.

Yet, in everything I have seen, I feel great pity for only one person – Rhoda. Although she had a traumatic brain injury, she could live a wonderful life if she chose to work in therapy to claim it. She simply refused to give herself the opportunity. And, on a deeper level than I think even she would admit, she refused to allow herself to feel hope.

I consider her the most broken of us all.

We either make ourselves miserable,
or we make ourselves happy.
The amount of work is the same.
~ Carlos Castaneda

The Champion

Cheryl was already a patient in the ABI unit when I arrived. She was in her early twenties and I considered her the most severely impaired of anyone. She was also severely physically injured and was in a wheelchair. She struggled to communicate in guttural sounding grunts. It was torture to watch this once vibrant young woman trapped in a wheelchair with a mind that still understood words spoken to her. She simply could not respond in any intelligible way. She had been the passenger in a car accident. I prayed that she had no memory of the wreck that had stolen so much from her young life.

Cheryl's arms and legs could not extend fully outward. Her hair was falling out. There were random clumps of thin short hair that lay on her shining scalp. She resembled a woman eighty years old. She appeared thin and frail, and so fragile that a strong wind could whisk her away. She always sat in the same far corner of the lunchroom. Her mother was there to assist her in eating. I am ashamed to admit that, after a while, I began to think of her as a fixture in the room, like a chair or table.

I made some half-hearted attempts to talk with her when we shared life skills therapy, but communication between us was rare. As the days progressed, I would speak, but not really listen for her response. I did not try to get to know her or to make any real effort to let her know that someone else, besides her Mom, prayed for her. This routine continued for a couple of weeks, until one afternoon I learned to see the heart of a true champion.

As with most of life's important lessons, my day started routinely. When it came time for physical therapy I realized that my therapist was absent. Cheryl's therapist would work with both of us for the hour. The therapist placed a simple tongue depressor in front of us. She explained that she was going to place one end between each of our fore fingers and thumbs. Neither of us was to let it slide out of our fingers as we simultaneously pulled against each other. We were to concentrate on holding on to the tongue depressor and pull when she said, "Go".

I was just deciding how I could beat Cheryl without making it look too easy when the therapist said, "Go!"

We both began to pull. It took about two seconds for Cheryl to snatch the tongue depressor from my finger and thumb. The therapist looked slyly at me, as if I had intentionally let Cheryl win, but I was as surprised as she was by the outcome. She set up the tongue depressor for round two. This time I managed to hold on for about five seconds. Each time we repeated this exercise, designed to strengthen our ability to grasp, we pulled longer and longer. Both of us had fiercely competitive spirits.

Towards the end of the hour, we were competing in a marathon of grasping and pulling. Beads of perspiration formed on my forehead from the exertion and concentration needed to hang on to that tongue depressor. With each competition, Cheryl became an even tougher competitor. Her determination to win each round fueled my desire to at least win one. I don't think either one of us even noticed the therapist except when she was putting the tongue depressor in our hands to start the next round. The world had shrunk to the two of us and the contest.

By the end of the hour, I think both of us were exhausted – I know I was. I had spent an entire hour pulling on a stupid tongue depressor until sweating, and I had not won one single round. Our last round seemed to last five minutes. Cheryl simply refused to quit, refused to lose even one time, refused to slack off. She was a true competitor.

As I looked into her face to congratulate her, I experienced a moment I hope to never forget. It was as if her heart had been cracked open, and I was allowed to feel the wonderful, powerful spirit of this young woman who would never give up. She didn't speak it, but it hung in the atmosphere and emanated from within her innermost being – pure power that could actually be felt. This awesome raw energy bore a hunger that dwelled deep within her heart. I felt awestruck.

I don't know how long I sat there looking at her. I glanced at the therapist. She too seemed awed by what had just happened. I knew that we had both felt the same thing. Neither of us spoke. Finally, I smiled at Cheryl. I complimented her on her tenacity. Slowly, with great effort, she raised her arm as high as she could. Painstakingly, her hand formed a fist.

What a champion!

Within the sorrow, there is grace.
When we come close to those things
that break us down, we touch those
things that also break us open.
~ Wayne Muller

Déjà vu

I wondered what I could say to Andy as I approached his room at Shepherd Center. Were there words to cheer my twenty-one year old cousin who had been paralyzed in a car accident? It was spring 1981, and as I neared his room, I put on a smile and hoped that the right words would be there. I opened the door and walked in.

He saw me and gave me a huge grin saying, "I'm so thankful I have my hands!" I have watched him at family gatherings searching for the chink in his armor, but he has never lost his genuine love of life and his amazing thankful attitude. Now, in a bizarre reciprocal déjà vu, he and his brother Danny had come to visit me at Shepherd Center twenty-four years later. As he held my hand I felt the deep calluses that had worked into his palms from days, weeks, months, years, decades of wheeling around in his chair. In all of that time he has been the essence of thankfulness and humor in our family. He would be surprised, and I hope pleased, to learn that I have always considered him the glue that binds our extended family closer together.

I have often wondered if Andy felt the same trepidation before entering my room at Shepherd Center that I had felt before I entered his room so long ago. Did he also search for words to cheer me up? If so, he needn't have worried. I had learned from the master.

Watching him live his life now for twenty-eight years has provided me the blueprint for a thankful life. Like him so long ago, I was determined that no one would visit me and leave feeling pity. I was too thankful for life, too thankful for hope, and so very thankful to be surrounded by such love from my family and friends that I couldn't feel down for long. Andy has taught me that the great key to living well is to live in thankfulness.

We talked recently about faith. He says his faith, his reliance on God, helped him remain positive about his long-term outcome. Then he told me something I hadn't considered.

"You know, Diane, God is not the only important component of overcoming tragedy. I have seen people of faith who could not. They allowed bitterness to grow in their heart and they were eventually defeated. Every person I have seen struggle hardest for health has either left God out of the struggle or has not engaged himself or herself in working for it. You are the other important part of healing. If you expect God to do it all, it won't get done. Don't underestimate your part in the hard work to reclaim your health."

I fought back tears as I thought of the wisdom learned from one so young, one who has endured so much.

Tragedy does not build character; it reveals it.
~ John Wooden (as adapted by Andy Lane)

The Boys

After completing a six-week stay at Shepherd, I was transferred to Pathways for six weeks of further inpatient treatment. That is how I found myself, a fifty-year-old mother of three teenagers, living in a dorm with seven guys.

My three teenagers were greatly amused at this latest development. They became fond of saying things like, "Okay, Mom, I don't want to hear any reports about you sneaking around after you're supposed to be in bed." Or "I'd better not hear about any loud partying." Of course, whoever said this always looked at the other two and all three would smirk.

I quickly learned that life in a dorm with seven brain-injured guys can border on the bizarre. Tim was by far my most unforgettable dorm mate. Like me, he had been injured in an auto wreck. Like me, he was also injured in a side impact on the drivers' side of his vehicle. A drunk driver ran a red light and struck him. I, on the other hand, had the dubious honor of pulling out in front of a truck while talking on my cell phone.

Not long after Tim arrived, he and I were watching the morning news on TV in the common room before going downstairs for breakfast. A consumer safety expert explained why car manufacturers should be reinforcing the doors of cars to better withstand a side impact crash. The shot cut to an automotive spokesman who quoted statistically low numbers for people injured in this type of crash. He further explained that there weren't enough of these crashes to justify the added expense consumers would pay to reinforce car doors. In fact, he assured the camera, he was willing to bet that his listeners wouldn't even know someone injured in this type of crash. Without speaking, and in unison, Tim and I looked at each other sitting in our wheelchairs. No words were necessary.

I remembered Tim as the guy with Velcro on his hand cast to attach a spoon to assist him in eating. When he arrived at Pathways, I took time to teach him the ropes. I helped him fill out his daily schedule, and showed him the Rubbermaid containers where he would store his dry goods. I explained that inpatients were scheduled to shop on Mondays at the local grocery store and returned to store their own personal food in the refrigerator. I explained the whole new routine.

Every morning we were awakened at 7:00 a.m. We bathed, dressed, made our beds, straightened up our rooms and went down to breakfast by 8:00 a.m. Once downstairs we performed as many tasks as we could physically perform to make our own breakfast. These tasks were made easier with needed items being easily accessible for wheelchair bound patients. I really enjoyed doing these tasks because it made me feel like I was regaining control of my life.

Tim always kept a close eye on me as I fixed my breakfast and lunch each day. If I ate Cheerios, then he ate Cheerios. If I made toasted waffles, then he made toasted waffles. It was the same with lunch. If I made a peanut butter and jelly sandwich, he had one too. One morning I craved a grilled cheese sandwich. Since this required use of the stove, and Tim was still unable to use the stove, I decided to grill two. When complete I added sliced tomatoes, cut them both identical, and set one plate down for Tim and the other and me.

He looked up and said, "You know, I really wanted a grilled cheese sandwich this morning, how did you guess?"

After breakfast we all set out for morning meeting in the therapy building. Morning meeting was a fifteen-minute meeting that stressed current events among other things. Tim was a fifty-year-old bachelor from South Georgia who had two cats he called his boys, and two sisters who visited regularly. On a recent visit one sister had given him a cell phone that he wore on a cord around his neck. We had just started morning meeting when Tim's phone rang loudly.

Our host, a therapist named Thomas, glanced over at Tim and continued to talk to us as Tim answered loudly saying, "Hello? Yes this is Tim. No you didn't interrupt anything. I'm just in morning meeting."

Thomas motioned for Tim go into the hall to talk. Tim didn't catch the cue because he continued to speak at full volume to a contractor he had hired to build a ramp up to his porch.

The contractor must have told Tim that one of his cats had come up on the porch. We heard him loudly say "Is it the orange one with white paws? Put the phone down to his ear."

Thomas made a valiant effort to continue to lead a discussion with the class, but it was a losing battle. I glanced around the room and saw that every other patient was doing what I was doing – listening to Tim.

"Hello big boy. Do you miss Daddy? You be a good boy and stay off of the porch and out of the man's way, okay?" he spoke loudly to the cat. By this time I noticed that even Thomas had stopped talking and was listening intently to the conversation. The contractor must have come back on the line because we heard Tim say, "Yes, that will be fine. Oh, will you do me a favor before you lock the house up? Leave a note in the kitchen for my sister. Tell her to fix the boys a grilled cheese sandwich today for lunch. I know there's plenty of cat food, but somehow I just know they'd really like that." He listened for a moment and then said, "No, you didn't interrupt anything at all. Call me anytime."

I looked at Thomas to see his reaction. I felt sure he would be annoyed with this loud and lengthy interruption. I was surprised to see his shoulders were bobbing slightly and his eyes were filled with tears. He was silently laughing. He tried to regain his composure and speak, but he just couldn't pull it off. We all shared this lighthearted laugh. I glanced at Tim and was pleased to see that he was laughing too.

As we left morning meeting for different therapies, I realized that my breakfast and lunch selections were causing consequences I hadn't expected. While in cognitive therapy class I thought about my upcoming lunch. During the next hour I shared the gym in the physical therapy room with Tim and several others, but I couldn't keep my eyes off of Tim. He was learning to use a walker. I thought about the morning's revelation. I had known that I was affecting Tim's personal menu selection. I wondered how long I had been making the dining choices for the boys. By lunchtime I knew exactly what I wanted for lunch.

I entered the lunchroom and wheeled directly to the pantry. I dug down into the bottom of my Rubbermaid container, hoping I still had a can left. I found one and then located a can opener. As I worked to open the can I glanced at Tim. He watched me intently. After opening the can I made two large tuna sandwiches, one for Tim, one for me. After all, I told myself with a smile of accomplishment, the boys deserved a treat for staying off of the porch and out of the contractor's way.

We can judge a man by his treatment of animals.
~Immanuel Kant

Playing the Hand You're Dealt

I had seen Mike earlier that day at morning meeting, a fifteen-minute class every patient attended. During morning meeting the headlines of the day were discussed, and we repeated the day and date back to our host. Each of us had been diagnosed with an acquired brain injury, and every day we repeated the day and date in English and in Spanish. Even though the reasons for our brain injuries were as diverse as we were, we all started every morning in the same way.

It could have been boring, but Mike, a fellow patient, kept up a steady banter on every topic in the headlines. His most noticeable feature was the shiny brown helmet he wore on his head at all times. His irreverent, dry sense of humor caused me to laugh out loud, and that is not a bad way to start your day. Needless to say, Mike and I became friends, but our first face-to-face meeting was, like many events in a brain-injured environment – bizarre.

I wheeled into the physical therapy gym and struggled onto a mat. Mike was already lying on the other side of the mat. He looked over and asked, "So, how long are you in for?"

"Six to eight weeks."

"How much time have you done?"

"Three and a half months, how about you?"

"I've done five months. When were you released?" he asked.

"I haven't been. I'm an inpatient here at Pathways,"

"I'm an outpatient. So, what are you in for?"

"Car wreck, and you?"

"Brain tumor that required surgery and caused a blood clot and a stroke," he stated flatly.

"That's too bad, is that why you have to wear the helmet?"

"Yeah, and I had to have a tracheotomy too," he proudly added.

"So did I."

I saw his eyes dart to my throat to see if the scar was there, and then he said, "Well, I had to be put on a ventilator."

"Yeah, so was I."

"Well, I was in a coma for a week in the intensive care unit (ICU)," he volunteered proudly.

"I was in an induced coma in medical surgical trauma (MST) for a month."

"Ha! ICU is more critical than MST, and an induced coma doesn't count!" he shot back.

"What do you mean an induced coma doesn't count? Anyway, a month is way more than a week, and MST and ICU are both critical care units." I was beginning to realize that this conversation had quickly deteriorated from off-the-wall to weird, but being both stubborn, and curious about how this would end, I wasn't about to give in.

"I'm in a wheelchair."

"Me too."

"I can't use my arm."

"Me too."

"Well, I have double vision," he smugly stated.

"I'm blind in my left eye." I couldn't hide the smile of victory. Blind definitely beats double vision any day of the week. He paused, as if reviewing the cards life had dealt him, seeking a trump to beat the hand I was learning to live with.

"My stroke caused me to lose the use of my leg," he stated flatly.

I was waiting for this opening. This was my ace in the hole. I had been saving my best card for this moment.

"Yeah, I broke my leg and had sixty other fractures in my body." I tried very hard not to sound like I was gloating. After all, no one likes a winner who gloats.

I should have known that he was hiding a trump card too. He quickly pulled it out and played it.

"Well, I have a shunt!"

I paused and then asked, "What is a shunt?"

This time it was he that couldn't hide his delighted smile of victory. "A shunt is in my head and drains the fluid that accumulates around my brain."

Yuck!! I did not know if this was true or not, but it sounded gross! I heard myself sigh out loud and said, "You win. That is so disgusting."

He settled back on the mat with a satisfied smile. Then he glanced over and we both shared a smile that quickly escalated into total abandonment as we roared with laughter. It was one of those laughs that lead to the giggles. Each time we looked at each other, we laughed, until both of us were wiping our eyes and holding our sides.

As our therapists approached, we overheard one say to the other, "One thing about these two is you'll never hear them complaining or talking about their problems." We looked at each other through tears of mirth, and fell into another round of helpless laughter.

It was only later that I thought about my colostomy, the paralysis in the left side of my face, and my hearing loss. I really had held the winning hand, but I had lost because Mike was a master at playing the hand he'd been dealt. He taught me a very important lesson that day, "A merry heart doeth good like a medicine…" Proverbs 17:22a.

Nine months later I stood in line with my daughter to check out. It was the first time in over a year that I had walked around in a store and although I was extremely tired, I was really proud of myself.

A young male cashier noticed my cane and asked, "What happened to you?"

"Oh, I was in a car wreck."

"Really? I had one last year, but my wreck was much worse than yours. I broke my leg and spent the night in the hospital."

My daughter looked up to see me smiling as I replied, "Wow, that's too bad."

As we walked to the car, she asked, "Why didn't you tell him about your wreck?"

She looked bewildered, but said nothing more when I told her, "Honey, he's no Mike. He doesn't hold the cards to sit at the table and play a hand with us."

> *Laughter gives us distance. It allows*
> *us to step back from an event,*
> *deal with it and then move on.*
> *~ Bob Newhart*

American Idol

It was the fourth season of American Idol, and my third roommate Donita was definitely a fan. She was an attractive petite college student whose car had been struck by a semi-truck. Miraculously, she had survived without any physical injury, but had sustained a traumatic brain injury. I didn't care for reality shows, but I could hear her TV through the curtain as the hopefuls tried out. Their voices were awful – so awful that they were amusing.

On the second night, I watched along with her. By the third week I was hopelessly hooked. One especially bad contestant insisted that he was talented. He told the judges that his entire family had told him that he was a great singer. Donita laughed when I commented that his entire family must be compulsive liars. Later at Pathways, I would remember this evening and cringe with my own embarrassing "Idol" moment.

Maybe it was that I had survived when the odds were so low and I was thrilled to still be living. Maybe it was because spring is such a wonderful time of renewal, of new beginnings. Maybe it was the combination of a brain injury, being completely nuts before that injury, combined with the first two reasons – whatever the reason I found myself in front of the entire Pathways staff and patients singing *Just My Imagination* by The Temptations.

It started so innocently. Music therapy was listed on my daily schedule and I located the correct room and met with Thomas, Pathways morning meeting host, and staff music therapist. Through my daily encounters with him in morning meeting, I had a great deal of respect for him. His patience, genuine enthusiasm, and love for us were obvious. Days that he wasn't there seemed to start wrong.

As I entered his room, he asked, "Diane, what musical instrument do you play?"

I hesitated and then answered, "None. I took a few months of piano lessons when I was kid, but that's all."

"Oh, okay. Then you have sung in a choir, or chorus, right? I'm guessing you are an alto."

This time my hesitation stretched a bit longer. "An alto? I don't know. I've never had a singing class."

I cringed inwardly when I thought of a time many years ago. I had been vacuuming the living room floor with headphones on. I had gotten carried away when one of my favorite songs had come on the radio and was singing into the nozzle end of the vacuum cleaner. I threw in a few dance steps and performed a perfect James Brown-like turn to see my husband Scott leaning against the wall in the hallway laughing. He was doubled over and tears rolled down his face.

When he could finally speak he said, "Diane, I'm not saying you can't sing, but when you got to that last chorus, the cat jumped off of the couch and ran out of the room."

Thomas must have read it in my face, because he rolled my wheelchair in front of a keyboard.

"What's one of your favorite all time songs?" he asked.

"*Just my Imagination,* by the Temptations."

He played the song and even began to teach me the keys on the keyboard.

A couple of days later Thomas told me that he was working on some entertainment for lunch and he'd decided to form a group comprised of patients to do a number. *Just My Imagination* would be the song, he asked if I was interested.

Immediately I told him, "No!" But later I thought about it. Isn't that what the old me would have done? I was a different person now. Life was so sweet, and I wasn't going to turn down a chance to do something new and daring. I saw Thomas later and told him that I would give it a try.

We met in the billiard room of the dorm and practiced. A patient named John was awesome on the keyboards and I tentatively sang a few bars of the song. It was amazing! Maybe it was the thirty plus years of singing this same song in the car, but I sounded pretty good. I was given the lead. There were three backup singers. An irony in life was that Donita was one of them. We practiced diligently. I even told my husband about our upcoming show. On the day of the concert, Thomas told me the location had been changed to the morning meeting room.

I began to panic when I heard the announcement over the speaker system inviting all patients, therapists, and staff into the room to hear our song. As John played the first few bars, I looked up to a sea of smiling faces, opened my mouth, and croaked out the first line. My hands sweated, my throat constricted, and the second line was even worse. It was the most terrible rendition of the song I had ever heard. Even the contestant on American Idol living with a family of compulsive liars sounded better. It was so horrible that I pictured myself on American Idol as the most awful Idol contestant ever!

I imagined Simon in his most deadpan English accent saying, "That was the most horrible rendition of that song I have ever heard. In fact, it doesn't take much imagination to see the Temptations on the phone right now hiring a hit man to ensure you never sing that song again."

Her voice in tune, her timing perfect, Donita's back up singing sounded great! After what seemed an eternity, the song ended. My hands sweated, and my face was flushed with embarrassment until I thought of the silver lining in the black cloud of short-term memory loss associated with brain injury. Most of the patients listening wouldn't even remember it tomorrow. By next week it would be long forgotten. Later, one of the staff complimented me on my performance.

"I was terrible," I said. I wondered privately if she was related to that family of compulsive liars.

However, I did learn one very important lesson from my performance. Getting a new lease on life does not ensure that your vocal cords signed a new contract.

A month later, I was in the midst of a fierce scrabble game in the leisure room, when Donita spelled the word "idol," she glanced at me and grinned slyly. I laughed out loud in real joy! Not at the memory of that truly awful performance, or because I was losing at scrabble. I realized that she still remembered the awful concert and was well on the road to recovery!

If you had lived 2,000 years ago and sung like that, I think they would have stoned you.
~ Simon Cowell on American Idol

The Early Days

Those of us who awaken out of a coma into a world of confusion have no idea of the stress, the pain, the long days and sleepless nights that our families and friends have endured. We don't understand the relief and the worry in the faces of those we love. They experienced the initial joy at the growing realization that we will live, but must also deal with the harsh reality that we have sustained a traumatic brain injury. No one can say with any assurance how we will be.

We slept while they made the decisions, and signed the forms for the lifesaving operations and alterations to our bodies. We slept while they bonded with strangers who shared the couches, chairs, and telephone in the waiting room. We slept when they called family and friends and set up prayer chains. They watched as some of those families were shepherded into the hospital chapel to face the news that their loved one did not make it. We slept while they learned to fear being called into the hospital chapel.

Years after my accident, my husband, Scott, shared his memory of a young girl injured in a horseback riding accident. She was in the ward with me, both of us in a coma. Scott and this young girl's father became friends in the endless days of waiting. After Scott came in to visit me, his friend was asked to go into the hospital chapel. Scott was in the trauma ward during a scheduled ten-minute visit with me when this young girl died. Her father, overcome with grief, climbed into her bed and held her for the last time crying the tears of a man whose heart and life were shattered.

Yet, her prognosis for survival had actually been better than mine. Internal bleeding and extremely high temperatures raged in my body. There was a moment of crisis when my family was called back to the hospital. They had only been gone twenty minutes and had just arrived at the hotel. While they hurried back, Scott was allowed to come into the trauma ward where he found me surrounded by doctors and nurses and the floor around me covered in blood. They were simultaneously working on me and taking me into emergency surgery and he was allowed to kiss my forehead before I was rushed away. My children, my brother and his wife were asked to join Scott in the hospital chapel. Why I survived, and this young girl of twelve, with her whole life ahead of her, did not, is something I will never understand.

Those hours in the hospital chapel had to be the hardest ordeal my husband and my children have ever faced. I believe it was at this very instant in time that I experienced the moment on the precipice described at the beginning of this book.

It is in these early days of the injury that the family suffers most. The patient is unaware of the turmoil and anguish of the family. It is only when the patient wakes that the family breathes a collective sigh of relief. This is when the patient begins to climb the slow and rocky path from suffering to healing.

It was five months after the car accident and I had finally been released to go home. I was still in a wheelchair and was a daily outpatient for therapy, but I was finally home. On my second weekend at home my husband insisted that I ride with him to Memorial

University Medical Center to visit the doctors and nurses, and the EMTs who had saved my life. I could not sit in a vehicle for a long period of time without experiencing terrible back pain. So he arranged a bed in the back seat of his crew cab truck and we set out for Savannah. The four-hour trip was not as painful traveling this way. I had made three large fruit baskets for the day and night shift doctors and nurses in the Medical Surgical Trauma (MST) ward, and for the EMTs in Rincon who had cut me out of my car and had administered the first medical care that initially saved my life.

Scott was adamant that we go back and personally thank these people for saving my life. Since I didn't remember any of them, and because I was still extremely nervous traveling in a vehicle, I felt less than enthusiastic about the trip. Those feelings quickly changed when we entered the medical surgical trauma ward. The staff looked up with questions in their faces, because they did not recognize me. When they saw Scott's face they immediately looked back at me and understood who I was. I thanked them for saving my life. I told them that I would now be able to see my daughter and youngest son graduate high school. Untold wonderful family events lie in store ahead of me. They had given me a great gift. One woman reached out and hugged me tightly with tears in her eyes. I assumed she was one of the nurses. After we left, Scott told me that she was one of the doctors who had worked to save me.

Scott felt disappointed that a certain young doctor was not there. He explained that this doctor had told him I would not survive. I think that one of Scott's main objectives in this visit was to prove to this young man that life and death defy logic. There is no textbook guarantee when dealing with matters of the human spirit.

47

He was also disappointed that an older nurse was not there. She had offered him that most precious of all commodities when facing the possibility of losing someone you love – hope.

After we left the hospital we traveled up the road to Rincon, a suburb of Savannah. We located the EMT building, but were disappointed to learn that the man and woman EMT team who saved me were off duty that day. We left them a fruit basket and a thank you card. Their supervisor and another EMT seemed surprised to learn that we had traveled four hours just to express a heartfelt thank you.

Going back and reminding people who work in jobs of life and death that they are appreciated is very important. They remember those they could not save. They need to be reminded that many of us live because of their efforts.

I think of the hundreds of people who have given their expertise to extend and improve my life and I feel so thankful. The doctors, nurses, EMTs, therapists, technicians, counselors, and many others have all worked to give me a full life. It is almost overwhelming when I consider the sum of their efforts on my behalf. None of us are self-made. All of us owe those who have helped us along the way. My list is longer than most, and therefore I feel my obligation is greater.

There are no guarantees in life. Life is this very moment. It is now. I feel a pressing need to spend it wisely. Once spent it cannot be retrieved. Let me always remember this.

We are not living in eternity. We have only this moment, sparkling like a star in our hand, and melting like a snowflake. Let us use it before it is too late.
~Marie Beyon Ray

There Aren't Enough Cheerleaders

It was a holiday week and few people were in the physical therapy gym. I lay on a mat with my right leg hooked up to electrodes programmed to shock for a minute and a half, and then rest for thirty seconds. I would lay here for fifteen minutes hoping that my leg would learn to wake up and feel sensation again. Then I saw him.

He wheeled himself into the gym. He struggled out of his chair, slowly raised himself, and stood. He was vertical! Only he knew what stamina, and resolve had sustained him. Only he knew the days, weeks, and months of pain and determination that had brought him to this moment in time.

His therapist held on to the gait belt fastened around his waist. Painstakingly he deliberately moved his right foot and then miraculously his left. His whole concentration commanded his feet to move. I watched in silence as he directed his mind and energy into this moment of time. Each step was carefully executed. It was as if he was at war – his mind determined to once again rule his body. He began to sweat with the demanding effort of the task. He used no walker, and no cane. He was *walking* with just his feet.

His therapist directed him to walk out one door, and return to the gym by the other door. As he went out of sight, I said a silent prayer that he would remain tough. I caught myself holding my breath in anticipation. It took several minutes for him to reappear. Gone was the man I had seen exiting the first door. The man entering the door was exhausted, and yet, in his eyes I noticed a light of excitement and hope. He was bathed in sweat, but his focus had not wavered. Finally, he reached his wheelchair. Slowly, steadily he lowered himself, as if savoring, memorizing this moment of triumph.

Then the most amazing thing happened within me. I fought within myself to squelch it, but like an erupting volcano, it would not be denied.

From the depths of my heart bubbled up a loud and victorious "Ta-Dah!" I felt my face grow warm with embarrassment.

He turned and laughed. "That is exactly what I was thinking."

What I had just witnessed had moved me beyond words. I am used to watching a healthy young man in the prime of life run down a football field and catch a football. If he scores a touchdown, many will cheer him. A squad of cheerleaders will perform back flips and somersaults to celebrate the event. Yet, the miracle that I had just witnessed had been performed in silence. A lone "Ta-Dah" had marked the event as worthy of recognition. It seemed sad that this triumph had not been as celebrated. Sometimes there just aren't enough cheerleaders in the world.

Later when I thought about what I had witnessed, I realized that God has known since the foundation of the world that we would need more cheerleaders. He already has a plan. Isn't that one of the tasks of angels?

"And suddenly there was with the angel a multitude of the heavenly host praising God and saying,

Glory to God in the highest, and on earth peace, good will toward men." Luke 2:13-14

Could my cheer earlier be the echo of some spiritual cheer of thanksgiving that only our spirits felt? The God who loves each of us enough to remember the number of hairs on our head surely celebrates our earthly victories. Wouldn't a man's first steps after relentless time spent in a wheelchair be worthy of an angelic high five?

Gratitude is our most direct line to God and the angels. If we take the time, no matter how crazy and troubled we feel, we can find something to be thankful for.
~ Terry Lynn Taylor

Kindness

He was young, he was handsome, and he was the victim of a gunshot wound to the head. He was a walking miracle. The gunshot scar above his right eyebrow was barely visible and was incapable of revealing his amazing, miraculous story.

He had a perfect smile of compassion and healing. He had a calm gentle manner that immediately put you at ease around him. He had been given an alias by Grady Memorial Hospital upon his arrival in the emergency room. It is standard procedure to provide all survivors of violent attacks an alias as protection if the perpetrator has not been apprehended.

I thought his alias was Robert Johnson. As he explained this to me I tried to imagine the person given the responsibility of doling out aliases. Was it a coincidence that his alias was the name of a legendary blues guitarist? Could I expect to be meeting a John Lee Hooker, John Hammond, or perhaps B. B. King next? I later learned that this was not his alias, but cannot remember the correct one. Remembering one name is hard enough for a TBI survivor, remembering two was hopeless.

I asked him the details of his gunshot and he explained that he was visiting his Mother during the Christmas holidays and had gone out with a neighbor to play golf. When he returned home he interrupted a burglary in progress. Entering his mom's house through the garage into the den he was approached by a man carrying a gun and was ordered to give up his wallet and car keys. He did as he was told. Sitting on the couch he looked up at the intruder who pointed the gun point blank at his head and fired.

The bullet was lodged on the left side of his neck. The bullet had miraculously done little damage. He did have trouble swallowing and the tracheotomy scar was still fresh on his throat. Other than that, he seemed in good health.

He shared a room with Houdini and two other patients. He was like a breath of fresh air for the ABI unit and I enjoyed his company immensely. Nothing rattled him. He seemed to always radiate tranquility, peace, and acceptance. In a place where all of us were broken in some way, he seemed the most whole to me.

Much later he would discover that he had an undiagnosed injury. His jaw had been broken and he would need to have corrective surgery. As time progressed the bullet began to work its way to the surface. He was scheduled for an outpatient procedure to remove the bullet. At our next group therapy meeting he shared that he had been shocked to learn that Novocain had to be administered in a shot. This handsome guy with perfect teeth had never had a cavity and thought that his neck area would be deadened with a cream. Those of us who had already undergone oral surgery to replace knocked-out teeth found his discovery deeply amusing.

I came to know him well during our time spent in Shepherd and Pathways. We shared physical therapy classes, group therapy (where I learned to finally remember his real name) and life skills classes.

He and I had said goodbye to many patients who had shared our lives when we were most fragile. He was my last link with a patient who had experienced Shepherd Center with me. As his release date from Pathways approached I became very apprehensive. He had become the one constant fixture in my new world of therapies, doctors, corrective surgeries, and the follow up therapies. He had been there with me through it all and had listened to every thought I shared in group therapy. He had been a gentle presence, an open ear, an understanding and calm spirit in a world turned upside down.

I didn't realize how emotionally attached I had become to this pleasant easygoing young man until his last day at Pathways. As I tried to tell him goodbye, I broke down into tears surprising both of us. I had said goodbye to many others – therapists and patients. Having him leave was the most emotional of them all. His quiet patience, his shared understanding of this world of rehabilitation, and his kind and gentle demeanor would leave a void that could not be filled.

None of us can comprehend the tremendous impact we have on others by simply offering acceptance and kindness. He taught me how powerful it is to simply be kind to someone else.

Kindness is gladdening the hearts of those who are traveling the dark journey with us.
~Henri-Frederic Amiel

What You Were

Designed to provide holistic healing, Shepherd Center and Pathways offered classes in recreational therapy, life skills, and group therapy as well as the more traditional occupational, cognitive skills, physical, and speech therapies. I began to paint in recreational therapy. Although I had no artistic talent, I thoroughly enjoyed it. During my second day of painting therapy, I realized for this moment, I was nearly pain free. It became the part of my week that I felt most peaceful. Looking back, I know that this one hour class, twice-a-week, helped to save me from depression.

Group therapy was another class that I would not have chosen to participate in. However, this class helped me understand that some of my feelings were universal and that I was not alone. Others had the same hopes and fears. We encouraged and we admonished each other as needed. As another patient said, "In here, we keep it real." It wasn't always pleasant, but it was always positive.

The therapists excelled in their knowledge and practical application, but there was one thing they could not know – what it felt like to face catastrophic loss.

And so it happened one morning in therapy that one of the newer therapists said to me, "Just remember one thing. You will never be what you were."

I had heard her say this to other patients and it always made me grit my teeth. She may have felt that she was helping patients and wanted them to have more realistic expectations of their future, but I interpreted this to mean that we were diminished and were all somehow less than we had been.

Before I could stop myself, I exploded, "You are absolutely right! I will never again be what I once was. Every person in this room, except you, has been tried by fire and we are still standing. I feel so much respect for all of us, because I understand what we have suffered and I understand the courage it has taken to get this far. You don't have a clue."

She was shocked by my outburst and before she could recover I went on, "Believe me, no one knows better than me that I am a different person. I am more sensitive, and I feel more sympathy for those who suffer." I saw her eyes begin to fill with tears as I continued, "I may have a brain injury, but I'm not crazy. No one would choose to look as I do right now. You are absolutely right! I will never, ever be the person I once was, because I believe that I am a better person today!" There was a sudden knock at the door and she went out into the hall to discuss an unrelated matter. While she was outside, I tried to get my emotions under control.

After experiencing a brain injury, outbursts such as mine are not uncommon. However, this was only the second one I had experienced and I was visibly shaking. I glanced around the room at my peers to see what the fallout might be from such a flare-up. Sitting in a wheelchair across the table was Marilyn. She understood what people said to her, but she was still learning to communicate and had a limited vocabulary.

She had tears in her eyes and she struggled to speak. She finally said, "dank ou."

I smiled at her. As I glanced around the table, I saw no judgmental looks from my peers, only smiles and acceptance. I was among friends.

The rest of the class was quiet. It was though we were all sitting in the eye of a hurricane that had just thundered through the room.

Finally, Frank, the prankster in the group, spoke up and said, "Feeling better are you? Got that off of your chest, did you? I guess we can be sure of one thing – none of us will ever be told that we will never be what we were again. So, when she comes back in here can we get on with therapy?"

I sheepishly glanced around the room and found a room full of grinning faces looking back. When she came back into the room we started again.

It is not the brains that matter most, but that
which guides them – the character,
the heart, generous qualities…
~ Fyodor Dostoyevsky

I Want To Go To Cincinnati

Pathways differed from Shepherd in several ways, but the most obvious were the inpatient trips into the community to eat dinner, go on field trips, and to shop for groceries. These field trips were planned to re-integrate patients back into society. I understood the reasoning behind these field trips into the community, because we all needed to begin to learn how to live in the outside world again.

Yet, there was a crusty old curmudgeon voice in my head at each venture out that always silently asked, "When will I ever be out again with two vans full of eight to ten people using wheelchairs, walkers and canes?" It always made me smile at the thought of how we all must look to others. Pushing the curmudgeon down, I went, and I always enjoyed myself immensely.

There are patients in rehab facilities that become legends among the other patients and staff. That is how I heard about Carl. Although Carl had come and gone before I was a patient at Pathways, I had already heard of him, and I always thought of him while on these excursions out. Every time he left Pathways, Carl would find a way to wander through the parking lot in search of his car. No one could convince him that he no longer owned a car and no longer had a driver's license for that matter.

Before coming to Pathways, Carl had been a successful radiologist in North Carolina. A brain tumor and the surgery to remove it had caused a brain injury and Carl was at Pathways to learn skills to once again live independently. He must have really loved his car, because he continued to search for it at every chance.

When he went out on the Monday afternoon trip to the supermarket to buy groceries for the week, Carl inevitably wandered through the parked cars. When walking from the therapy building to the dormitory, Carl detoured through the shared parking lot always searching for his car. After a field trip at dinner, as he made his way to the vans, he searched left and right at the cars parked in the lot.

When not searching for his car, he would sometimes write prescriptions on notebook paper. His experience in the medical field served him well and he understood the medical jargon everyone was exposed to every day. He was a most helpful translator to patients when needed, and enjoyed being around people. Carl was fun and he lifted the spirits of those around him.

The ratio of men to women in the dorm during his stay was the same as it was for me, all guys with one girl. This lone female in the dorm was far away from her home in Ohio. Because of the distance, she rarely had visitors and had become quite homesick. She functioned fine during daily therapy when things were busy, but would get homesick and moody in the evening. She missed her friends and family. Her homesick attitude finally exploded one night.

It was two in the morning when she began yelling in the hallway. She had gotten out of bed and she was loudly calling out over and over, "I want to go to Cincinnati." Each time she said it she increased the volume in her voice. As the staff tried to quiet her down she reached a fevered pitch, and breathing in deeply she yelled at the top of her voice, "I want to go to Cincinnati!"

Suddenly, from a darkened dorm room down the hall came Carl's sleepy, irritated voice, yelling loudly in reply, "If I could find my damn car, I would drive you there myself!"

At times of the severest depression, humor is what binds people together.
~ Robert Carlyle

Bug-Eyed Sunglasses

As I was waiting for my physical therapist, I remembered a day from years ago I have always referred to as my rainbow day. That day had started as a bad day when I had overslept causing me to face rush hour traffic in Atlanta. It had continued on with various mishaps occurring all day long. Murphy's Law would have given an approving nod to that day.

Finally, after what seemed an eternity I was heading home from work. Although it was still sunny, it began to rain, and with the rain came the inevitable traffic slow down. Living west of Atlanta always kept the sun in my face, and as I reached for my sunglasses I noticed they were missing. I had left them at home. I quickly glanced at the passenger sun visor and found a pair of sunglasses that someone had left behind. I put them on and looked into the mirror. These sunglasses were huge and gave me the appearance of a giant fly, but they were better than nothing. This is a perfectly rotten ending to a perfectly rotten day, I thought grumpily.

Then I looked up and saw the most brilliant rainbow I have ever seen. It arched right over the road. It wasn't a small faded rainbow. It was enormous. The colors were brilliant and dazzling, with each color fully and gloriously distinguishable; iridescent red, orange, yellow, green, blue, indigo, and violet that gleamed in the sunlight. It appeared as though at any moment I would be driving right through it and I wondered how it might feel to be illuminated by with the myriad colors of the rainbow.

I marveled at how I had not seen it before and moved the sunglasses further down on my nose. It was not visible without the bug-eyed sunglasses. I had to smile. God really does have a great sense of humor. He placed the rainbow in the sky to remind us that he keeps his promises. Although things were not going smoothly that day, I was reminded that God was still with me, and still in control.

Going through physical therapy with so many broken bones still trying to mend was an exercise in pain and fear I have never experienced before, and I hope to never experience again. Thinking back to the rainbow day, I realized that I had no concept of what a bad day was back then. I had been facing a series of trivial events, in comparison to the challenges I was now facing. From this new perspective, I thought of all of the countless days in my past when I had allowed minor inconveniences to rob me of the simple pleasure of enjoying life.

However, one lesson that I learned on the rainbow day was now a daily reality. I knew that even though I may not see the rainbow, it was still here. God, who always keeps his promises, was here with me to give me the strength to continue on. Knowing he was with me made everything I was going through tolerable.

In that moment I made a promise to myself. From now on when I felt despair, I would try to imagine myself putting on an invisible pair of those bug-eyed sunglasses. I would mentally re-create the experience of those glorious colors again, and remind myself that I was not alone. I could conquer this. I could do it. God still sits on the throne, and I could endure.

> *God will be present, whether asked or not.*
> *~ Latin Proverb*

Ice Chips

My brother Doug was a frequent visitor at Shepherd Center. Late one afternoon he dropped in and we had a long talk. He reminisced about my time spent in Savannah. When I came out of the coma, he took a week off work and drove to Savannah to spend every day in the hospital with me. He asked if I remembered the day that he talked with me all afternoon and fed me ice chips. When I told him no, I saw the look of disappointment on his face.

I felt bad, but couldn't think of anything appropriate to say, so I let it drop. I had the feeling that our time together had been significant. I wanted to tell him that just because I didn't remember it, didn't mean that I hadn't also been moved at this special time during that day. The loss of memory by one person does not undo the love given by another. I wanted to say something to him to make him feel better, but I couldn't fit the thoughts and words together.

Five months later when I met Chris, I would begin to understand how Doug felt. I first saw Chris during my last week at Shepherd Center before being transferred to Pathways. He was from South Carolina, and had a lovely young wife and a new baby. He had been injured in a fall on a construction job. The height from which he had fallen would have killed most men.

Somehow he had survived. Seeing him so severely damaged in that huge chair broke my heart.

He was in the largest wheelchair that I had ever seen. It was motorized and his arms and legs had to be secured to the chair. He was a tall and burly young man who could not yet speak. One morning I saw his leg break free from a restraining strap, and it twitched uncontrollably until a tech secured it back in position. I considered Chris the most injured living person I had ever seen. After spending eleven weeks in catastrophic care hospitals that is saying something.

The following week I was transferred to Pathways. Many months later I limped down the hall with a cane when the elevator doors opened. Chris wheeled himself out. He was pushing himself in a standard sized chair and he was talking to his therapist.

I leaned down and said, "It is so exciting to see you looking so good." He had no idea who I was and his face showed it. I told him that I had been at Shepherd when he first came in and that he looked fantastic. He seemed pleased, but also nervous that this woman he didn't know was making such a fuss about him.

Two weeks later I arrived for therapy a half hour early. I decided to wait in the leisure room. The leisure room was designed for patients' comfort and included magazines, games, and a computer for patients to use. It was a place for patients to relax between therapies or was sometimes built into a patient's schedule for playing games with other patients.

As I entered the room I saw Chris stretched out on the couch. One glance at him told me that he was having a very bad day. I reintroduced myself and we started to talk. He had just learned that a very good friend had died and he was physically unable to make the trip to South Carolina for the funeral. He was feeling pretty useless and vulnerable. As he and I began to talk I could tell that he was beginning to feel better. After twenty-five minutes I had to leave for therapy. Chris was sitting up and smiling. He asked my name again and he told me he was really glad that we had talked. As I left, I felt good about being able to cheer him up.

Two days later, I saw him in the hall. I smiled and said, "Hi Chris, how are you doing today?"

He looked at me with a blank expression and said, "I'm fine."

It was obvious that he didn't know who I was, nor did he remember our conversation of two days ago. I felt disappointed that he didn't remember the special conversation that helped him through his bad day.

Like those ice chips from Doug, the event had melted into the recesses of a damaged mind. I began to understand the frustration of those living with a TBI survivor. I had experienced how disappointing it was for my brother that I couldn't remember how he had helped me get through a bad day, and the loving moments we had shared. That is the real tragedy of traumatic brain injury. It is not the time lost in a coma, but events lost in the mind. Maybe when Doug reads this he will finally understand.

The ones who count are those persons who – though they may be of little renown – respond to and are responsible for the continuation of the living spirit.
~Martin Buber

The Proper Motivation

Joe was one of my dorm mates and was admitted on the same day that I arrived at Pathways. He was learning to transition from a walker to a cane when I met him.

He had been driving a company pick-up truck on a major four lane road with a grassy median when a drunk driver drove off of the road, became airborne on the higher elevated grassy median, and crashed through the roof of his truck cutting his vehicle in half and critically injuring Joe. The drunk driver escaped injury. In his car was a case of empty beer cans. He had spent twenty-four hours in jail and had promptly bonded out. He had disappeared leaving a wide path of human suffering behind. His family claimed to have no knowledge of his present address.

Joe had a wife and three young children. He and his wife also cared for both sets of their parents. They were supposed to have closed on a large home that would have given everyone the extra room needed to live together comfortably, but the mortgage company had cancelled the contract after discovering the news of Joe's physical injuries and his traumatic brain injury.

Joe's wife was a nurse and immediately recognized the challenges he faced with a traumatic brain injury. It took some time, but his wife, with help from his doctor, had finally convinced him that he would never be able to perform his old job. However, he remained optimistic about his life and left Pathways full of excitement with the prospect of his new role.

His wife was returning to work full-time and Joe would now be the primary caregiver to their elementary school aged children. He wanted to find another house large enough to care for their parents. I often wonder how he made out with his new life. I think he had the tenacity to pull it off. His brain injury would not stop this dad from being an important part of the family. Although he and his wife had now switched roles, which would certainly change the family dynamics, I have no doubt that they made it work. An occupational therapist was helping him learn to cook when he was released. The only outward appearance of any damage from his accident was that he now walked with a slight limp.

When I think of him I always smile. At breakfast one morning he had complained loudly to all of us sitting at his table about a therapy class on his schedule. He hated the class and had tried unsuccessfully to get out of it. He hated the repetition of all of the exercises. I looked at his schedule and made a mental note to go by while he was in therapy. I wheeled down the hall and glanced into his class. He was in the back of the room doing exercises looking like he hated every minute of it. On a lark, I slowed until only he could see me outside in the hall. When he glanced out, I smiled, and then, acting on impulse gave him the finger. His expression was priceless! His face changed from disgust at exercising, to stunned disbelief in a split second. I continued on down the hall chuckling loudly.

Maybe it was a guilty conscience, or maybe it was a survival instinct that caused me to turn and look behind. There, with his brand new cane, came a red-faced Joe hobbling wildly up the hall. Only he wasn't using his shiny new cane to walk. He wobbled up the hall as fast as he could manage and was silently shaking that shiny cane high in the air at me. I didn't look down to see if my wheelchair wheels left rubber marks on the carpet when I scratched off, but they should have.

Fortunately, I had learned to move pretty fast on my wheels. No one else witnessed this brief incident of road rage, but I am sure that any therapist would have been amazed that Joe could already walk without the use of a cane. They just didn't understand how to properly motivate him. I decided to keep this knowledge to myself.

Laughter and tears are both responses
to frustration and exhaustion…I myself
prefer to laugh, since there is less
cleaning up to do afterward.
~ Kurt Vonnegut, Jr.

When the Saints Go Marching In

I sat in my wheelchair waiting to go downstairs to the welcome party. My friend, Diane, had helped me decorate my wheelchair. My wheels were lined with lights that wound around each spoke in the wheels. Two batteries to power the lights were taped unseen with black electrical tape on the inside hub of each wheel. Above the backrest on each side were long wooden dowels that held a huge Mardi Gras banner approximately two foot wide above my head. Shiny purple, green, and gold streamers trailed the banner on each side. Scott had been sitting on the bed in the hotel room watching as Diane decorated my chair. He would smile and then shake his head at the sight of my wheelchair.

I was in Mobile, Alabama, the birthplace of Mardi Gras, in mid-April. I was registered for the National Association of Women in Construction (NAWIC) Region 2 Forum, an annual regional conference of women employed in the construction industry from Alabama, Georgia, and east Tennessee. I hadn't seen many of my friends in NAWIC in over six months, and I was terrified. What if I went downstairs and everyone felt sorry for me?

When the registration email for Forum had arrived in February, I really wanted to go, but I was terrified at the thought of going. I was still an outpatient at Pathways, but the conference was on the weekend. Scott seemed to intuitively know that I needed to go. I needed to learn to live again. He and my friend Diane had planned the trip. We went in Diane's SUV. She had driven while Scott and I sat in the back, surrounded by mounds of pillows to make the trip more comfortable for me. Although Diane and Scott had worked out the travel details, the wheelchair decorations were my idea.

I was hoping that my friends would see this as a sign that I was still me. I may look different and I may even act different, but I didn't want pity. I wanted to be accepted as me. A few minutes before seven Scott pushed my wheelchair to the elevator and we started down to the ballroom for the welcome party. I was excited, but also close to having a panic attack. Scott tried to calm me as we made our way down. As the elevator doors opened I saw my friends dressed in Mardi Gras gowns and masks waiting to enter the ballroom. They were planning to enter throwing beads to many who were already sitting inside at tables. Scott began to push my chair towards them and suddenly I found myself engulfed in a sea of love. My friends rushed over to hug me and make me feel welcome. Immediately my fears were dissolved.

As one friend, Anne, pushed my wheelchair closer to the door, I realized that I would be leading this group inside. To my delight, I had become the Mardi Gras float. In my lap were piles of Mardi Gras beads to throw.

An instant before the door opened I noticed that Scott was gone. Almost like a young child who suddenly misses a parent, I searched frantically in the crowd to

71

see him. I spied him leaning against the back wall next to a huge palm tree. He was smiling at me and tears were streaming down his face.

True friendship is seen through the heart not through the eyes. ~ Unknown

The Real World

Life in a catastrophic environment is sterile and pared down to the essentials. No energy remains to put on pretense. As one of the other patients aptly defined it – *it is what it is*. Long after my friends at Shepherd and Pathways had left I was still attending outpatient therapy. I had a brain injury, but also had other major physical ailments that required continual therapy well past nine months. I still had not been cleared to drive. During this time, I left the house only for therapy, doctor visits, and weekly grocery shopping. I never imagined that this extended time of isolation from the outside environment would have such a profound impact on me.

My first clue that I had become alienated from the outside world came as I sat in the waiting room of my oral surgeon to have implant surgery replacing the teeth knocked out in the wreck. Sharing the waiting room with me were two women in their thirties. They were in the middle of a conversation about their teeth.
I heard one woman say, "But I just don't like this tint of white, so I am going to have them replaced."

As their conversation continued, the door to the waiting room opened. A woman in a motorized wheelchair entered and parked herself into a very tight niche on the first try. We were both veterans of having our mettle tested and we felt an instant kinship.

She had also been a patient at Shepherd Center, and we began to talk. I found it interesting that patients in the spinal cord unit felt the same as many of us in the acquired brain injury unit.

Each of us looked into the other unit and thought, "At least I am not in that unit; it would be terrible to never walk again." Or "At least I'm not in that unit; it would be terrible to lose your ability to think clearly, your memory, or speech."

We smiled at each other knowing we both felt the other was worse off. We recognized in each other a steely resolve that survivors of catastrophe share.

After I had returned home, I thought about that overheard conversation in the waiting room. There was an uncomfortable feeling in the back of my mind, but I couldn't put my finger on it. I thought of those who have fought so hard to regain lost muscle, to rebuild strength to help them navigate wheels instead of legs, to regain some control in their lives, and maybe, to regain their independence. I thought of the raw courage in the daily fight to overcome pain and fear that I had observed in the ABI unit. I thought of the people who have left indelible imprints in my heart and mind, of the miraculous healing I have witnessed in this incomparable group of survivors. I wondered how many of the people I was now seeing, could handle enormous personal tragedy with the grace and tenacity that I had witnessed?

The uncomfortable feeling that I had been trying to define finally made sense, and I began to understand that I was looking at the 'real' world. I was seeing it clearly for the first time. I was looking at America, at all of the materialistic snares that abound from being the richest society on the globe. In my new encounters with people outside of the hospital environment, I was seeing a mirror image of how I used be. For the first time in my life, I saw myself as I was. It was hard to face. Although I would never have been able to see it or admit it then, I had been too materialistic. I realized that I was a mere shadow of the woman I have become.

I remembered a story I once heard about a group of Russian Christians that had been sponsored by an American church to come to America for a visit. Their hosts kept them busy seeing as much as possible about American life.

When it was time for them to leave, one of the church members told one of the visitors, "I will keep all of you in my prayers. You have so little in your country."

The guest replied, "In times of need it is easier to trust God. I will pray for Christians in America to be able to avoid the snare of materialism that is so prevalent here."

Which world is the real world? I thought about the rehabilitative therapy environment, the daily war of mind and body to regenerate and build a life from the ashes of catastrophic loss. I considered the world of reality shows, tinted white teeth, and the rampant consumerism that drives us. This illusion of 'real' permeates our culture distracting us from what is actually real. Television tells us that a survivor is someone placed on an island with a group of people. These people plot and scheme, build and break alliances, and could win a million dollars if left standing at the end. Integrity and courage are not necessary, and can even be obstacles to winning.

Ask a survivor of a catastrophic injury or illness what qualities helped them in their fight to survive. Ask this person from where they derived their strength.

Finally, ask them what is most important to them today. And begin to understand what is real.

And now abideth faith, hope and charity, these three; but the greatest of these is charity. ~1 Corinthians 13:3

Nip It

I knew that it was not uncommon for patients who had sustained a head injury to experience anger issues. I had seen other patients become extremely angry. I had even had a couple of episodes of anger myself. However, those two incidents did not cause me to recognize that I had anger issues. I do remember one time when Scott came to see me at Shepherd. He told me something one of our teenagers at home had done. Without even realizing that I was doing it, I had raised my arms and had shaken my hands. This gesture can best be described as a combination of hallelujah praise, and the robot on the old TV show, *Lost in Space,* with hands moving. Only I did not say, "Warning Will Robinson."

I didn't even realize that I was doing it. I didn't understand that this was my new of way of reacting to an overload of information and the ensuing anger.

My husband of twenty-eight years looked at me the first time I did it and said, "That's cute. I've never seen you do that before."

I didn't know what he was talking about until I realized what my hands and arms were doing. Once I came home this became my signature gesture right before I blew my top. He never commented that it was cute again. This gesture, like steam that issues from a volcano shortly before it explodes, signaled I was about to explode. Most of the time I never even realized I was doing it.

It is amazing how oblivious a person with TBI can be to the changes in their behavior. The instrument used to obtain accurate data has been damaged, and information retrieved is inaccurate, or unable to be retrieved at all. It seemed to me, in those days, that everyone asked me how I was doing. I remember feeling so frustrated at this question. Sometimes I just wanted to scream, "How should I know? I can't even remember what my house looks like or how to get there. You have the test results, you take blood every day, and you can read my charts. Why don't you tell me, and then we'll both know." As time went by, I began to remember these things, and I began to tell myself that I was fine.

When I was released from the hospital five months after my accident, I still thought I was managing fine, until my daughter came into my room one day.

"Mom, I want to talk with you about something important."

"Sure," I replied. "What's on your mind?"

She took a deep breath and then said, "I don't think you realize it, but you are yelling at Kacy a lot lately. You were just yelling at him a few minutes ago, and you are hurting his feelings."

This statement really shook me. I had always prided myself on being a supportive mom. Was I becoming a screaming parent without even realizing it? After she left my room I thought about what she had said. I had never seen myself as someone who had anger issues. At first I was overcome with guilt and cried. Then I began to think of how I could repair the hurt my son must be feeling. I thought and prayed through the evening about this anger. If I didn't know I was even doing it how was I to stop?

The next morning Kacy got up and went to school. He hadn't even told me goodbye. As the day wore on, I began to think of a plan. I waited eagerly for him to come home from school. Finally, I heard him come into the house and called him into my room. I noticed that he stood in the doorway. I wondered if my anger toward him had been so bad that he no longer wanted to be in the same room with me.

I began, "Kelly told me that I have been yelling at you a lot lately. First, I want to tell you how sorry I am for anything I have said to you that has hurt your feelings."

He quickly cut in, "Don't worry about it mom," and turned to leave the room.

"Wait a minute," I hurriedly added, "I think I have a plan to stop doing this."

He turned around and walked a few steps into the room asking, "What do you mean?"

"I was thinking that maybe you and I should have a code."

He looked intrigued and took a few steps more into the room asking, "A code?"

"Yeah, a code word to help me control my temper. If we have a code word you can say to me when you see that I am beginning to lose my temper I promise to shut up immediately."

He looked thoughtful as he walked over to the chair next to my bed and sat down. "What is the code word?"

"I thought that you should think of the word. What do you think?"

He was quiet for a minute and then said, "Nip it."

"Nip it?" I repeated back.

"Yeah." He smiled for the first time. "It's short for nip it in the bud."

"Okay then. That is settled. Now there are two rules we need to discuss."

I saw his smile fade as he asked warily, "What rules?"

"Well, the first rule is that you can only use the code when I am starting to lose my temper. After all, when you use the code word you are acting like the parent and I am acting like the child. For this to work, you can't abuse the code word."

He smiled again, and looked thoughtful and pleased at this statement as he said, "Okay."

"The second rule is that you can't tell anyone else about the code. This is strictly between us." He sat in the chair eyeing me for a moment, and then he leaned over and gave me a long hug. As he got up to leave he said, "Okay mom, we have a deal."

Over the next few days I tried to monitor myself closely and Kacy didn't have to use the code word. However, it was less than a week later and we were both in the kitchen when Kacy looked at me and said, "Nip it, Mom." I stopped talking immediately. After he left the kitchen, I thought about our conversation prior to the code enforcement and realized that I had been about to lose my temper.

Over the next few months Kacy used the code many times, and each time I cut off what I was saying and then tried to think of what had caused the code enforcement to be used. I was trying to learn not to do it again. By the third month Kacy rarely had to use the code. I was learning to manage my anger. As time went by I realized that it had been months since the code had been enforced. Our code had started as a secret, but others in the family had noticed that something was definitely going on.

When they asked about it I had replied that, "Kacy and I have a code."

This statement was met with blank faces, but no one asked me anything else. However, this quiet acceptance didn't mean that they weren't asking Kacy.

It was a Saturday morning and I had heatedly reminded my husband that I could not bend easily to pick up his socks on the floor. He would have to do this himself. I had retreated into the office and was typing on my computer.

It was about twenty minutes later when I heard Scott and Kacy talking. They were at the end of the hall, and I heard Scott ask Kacy, "What's the code word?" Apparently he had learned about the code, but did not know the words. Kacy has always been the funny bone in our family and I listened closely to hear his reply.

"Sorry, Dad, but code words only work with kids. I'm pretty sure that there is fine print on the bottom of every marriage license that renders code words null and void. That's what Mom said anyway." I heard my husband groan as Kacy gave a lighthearted laugh.

Anger makes you smaller, while forgiveness forces you to grow beyond what you were.
~ Cherie Carter-Scott

The No Lady

I had a conversation with Ruby the day before she was released from Pathways. She was in the gym getting her exercise schedule from her therapist. This would be her therapy routine when she returned home. I had seen Ruby in the hallways, but had never spoken to her.

I was surprised to learn that she was from Massachusetts, and I had to ask, "How did you hear about Pathways in Atlanta?"

"The No Lady told my husband Tom about Shepherd and Shepherd Pathways in Atlanta." She smiled when she saw the puzzled look on my face.

"Who or what is the No Lady?"

As her therapist made copies of her exercises, she filled me in on the No Lady. "I had a stroke over a year ago and was confined to a wheelchair. Each time my husband Tom tried to acquire the equipment I needed he would have to call our insurance provider. Each time he called he spoke to the same lady. Every time he spoke to her she would tell him no, the insurance policy did not cover a wheel chair, or whatever I needed. And each time Tom would read the policy to her over the phone pointing out that the policy did indeed cover whatever was needed. The No Lady's reply was always the same. Let me check with my supervisor for approval."

"Eventually I would get what I needed and what my insurance policy had stated was appropriate, but each time it was a struggle with the No lady. Over time Tom has become a layman expert in the provisions of my insurance policy, and with talking to the No lady."

"One day as Tom spoke with the No lady, she mentioned that Pathways in Atlanta had a great reputation for helping people with my medical challenges. She asked Tom if he might be interested in looking into a program like this. After some research and help from the No lady, we relocated temporarily in Atlanta for me to receive the cutting edge care that Pathways has provided."

Now, eight weeks later, she walked with a cane and a small leg brace and was looking forward to returning home to be closer to her children and grandchildren.

She concluded, "Isn't it ironic that the No Lady ended up being the person who helped us the most in the end?"

I thought about what she said and I realized that something very similar had happened to me. A woman I worked with had the reputation of being very aloof to coworkers. I always considered it typical workplace irony that she worked in our company's Human Resources department. Five months after my wreck, and the day after I was released as an in-patient at Pathways, my friend, Diane, drove me to my job to visit my friends.

As I wheeled into the lobby of our office building, this woman was the first person I saw. She came over and hugged me very tightly, and when she moved away she was crying. I was shocked! This woman that I would have sworn was the Ice Queen incarnate had been moved to tears. Throughout the entire healing process, she had ensured my insurance issues were handled. She had taken care of all of the paperwork keeping me and my family covered. She had been the person I learned to lean on for help, and she had always followed through. Like the No lady, I had not expected her to be the person who helped me the most.

I looked back at Ruby as she was now talking about a new patient that she and her husband had met a couple of nights ago. She and Tom lived in the apartments made available for patients and a family member in the outpatient program. They had run into a man from New England whose wife was a patient at Shepherd Center. They had gone with him to visit her and had all formed an instant bond.

"What's your new friend's name?"

"Oh, her name is Emily, but Tom and I just call her the Maine lady."

"Of course, she is from Maine?"

"Right," she agreed.

"I imagine you are you excited about leaving and seeing your children and grandchildren again," I said.

"Yes we are," then she elaborated, "Tom is going to call his sister tonight and tell her to meet us at the airport and to start praying for the Maine Lady." She explained that his sister was a devout Christian and they always made sure she prayed for things important to them.

"Her name is Linda, but we've always just called her ….

I cut her off and said, "No! Let me guess! It's the Christian lady, right?"

"Don't be silly. We wouldn't call her that. We call her the Prayer Lady."

I should have known.

Never judge. The heart of a man is so delicate so complex only its Maker can know it. Each heart is so different, actuated by different motives, controlled by different circumstances, influenced by different sufferings. ~ Anonymous

Iron Sharpens Iron

Two weeks after I arrived at Pathways my hair started to fall out. At first I noticed hair on my clothes and on the back of my wheelchair. Then after my shower I started having to brush my hair over a trashcan. When my bathtub drain clogged up I became really concerned. I have always had very thick hair and I could tell that my hair was becoming much thinner. I began to dread brushing it.

The nurse at Pathways explained this to me. "Sometimes the stress of a catastrophic event causes a patient to lose their hair or to break out with a bad case of acne."

My hair falling out was the final straw. I felt that I had lost control of absolutely everything in my life. During his evening visit, Scott responded with a combination wince and smile when I told him, "I always thought we would grow old together, but I never dreamed we would grow bald together."

The following morning as I brushed my hair, several large clumps came out and my scalp was now visible. I prayed, "God, if there is a lesson I need to learn from my hair falling out, or if there is a reason I must lose my hair, I ask you to give me the strength to bear this because I can't handle any more loss."

It was only after I finished my prayer and I touched my face that I realized I was crying. Later that day I spoke with my recreational therapist. She made arrangements to take me to have my hair cut very short. This was one way I tried to regain control. If my hair was going to fall out, then cutting it short would make it easier to bear.

Later, I thought about my prayer. I realized how much I had grown spiritually. Before my accident, I would have prayed, "God, I thank you for my hair not falling out. Amen." I would not have acknowledged that there might be a reason, or a lesson to be learned from this experience. I would have simply prayed a prayer telling God what I wanted him to do. I realized that I had reached a point in my walk with God that I really meant not my will, but thy will be done. It felt peaceful and exhilarating to be able to trust God so completely.

Five months later I was still an outpatient at Pathways and my hair was growing back extremely thick and wavy. I was surprised that the short haircut I now wore was a good look for me and I discovered that I really liked it. My physical therapist, Trish, had been a rock for me throughout the ordeal of losing my hair. She never showed a glimpse of pity, just the same tough work ethic, with a few irreverent barbs thrown in to lighten my heart.

Trish was an attractive, petite, ball of fire. She rode a Harley motorcycle, kick boxed, worked out in a gym, and ran for pleasure. She stood five foot three inches tall and weighed a hundred pounds soaking wet, but she was human dynamite. She kept all of us on our toes, both literally and figuratively. During my hour of therapy with her, I worked harder, sweated more, tried my best, dug down deep, laughed often, cried some, talked too much, and learned to walk! She had taken me from wheelchair, to walker, to cane and was working with me to navigate on a leg brace.

Though we were closer than the typical therapist/patient relationship, I was surprised when she called me at home one afternoon. "Diane, I wanted to tell you that I have been diagnosed with breast cancer. I have already had surgery and will be having chemotherapy over the next couple of months." I was stunned and asked, "How can I help you, Trish?"

A conversation began that included strategies for dealing with losing your hair and ended with a discussion on how to trust God and rely on him during times of great trouble. I shared with her my favorite scriptural verse that I used to give me strength and to help me overcome fear. "God is our refuge and strength, a very present help in trouble. Therefore we will not fear though the earth be removed, and though the mountains be carried into the midst of sea." Psalms 46: 1-2

During the next couple of months as Trish went through her chemotherapy treatments, I was there to witness her courageous fight. She never missed a day of work, and she kept that same tough spark that made her such a good therapist. As her hair began to fall out she cut it short, and then had a wig made that matched her cut. Eventually, she shaved her head. I had been expecting this. Trish would want to feel in control of her life. Eliminating the hair she couldn't control, gave her the mastery of her body again.

I kept Trish close in my prayers and she did the same for me. It comforted me to know that my friend not only gave me her best in skill and knowledge, but prayed for me as well. One day in therapy Trish told me that her husband had accepted a job in Texas. She would be leaving to join him in a couple of weeks. As we talked about this, I realized that we had become more than therapist and patient. We had become "sisters in surviving."

We kept each other strong and had made the other physically, mentally, and spiritually sharper. Though we were from the South, we were no longer steel magnolias– we were titanium! And so between us we devised the only plan that made sense. We would do a *Thelma and Louise*. In the movie Thelma and Louise drove off of a cliff holding hands. We decided on a more sensible end. We would leave Pathways at the same time. Maybe not as spectacular an ending as in the movie, but my experience at Shepherd had taught me that real life is always more miraculous than it is in movies. Our ending would not need special effects, and it gave us the option for continuing our personal journeys to the next stage wherever they led.

It was bittersweet to say our goodbyes. I remember thinking that this must be how soldiers in battle feel, to have to say goodbye to friends who have shared their peril. These bonds are forged with grit and courage summoned from the depths of your heart when most needed. They are sealed with the taste of your own salted tears, and with the knowledge that you have made a stand, have summoned the fortitude to face this goliath, and have endured.

Your heart opens wide to every experience, but the fabric of your mind is forever sheathed with unbreakable covering, like Excalibur sealed in stone. You are victorious! It is hard to let go of those who were essential to you in this battle. It is hard to allow them to leave you to pursue the next phase of their own journey. I discovered that there are no adequate words to say goodbye to someone who has shared these circumstances.

What is within your heart cannot be uttered into words. In your heart these emotions are as deep and vast as the sea. Expressed in words they become stiff and small. There are no words to describe the experience of sharing such a significant part of our healing journey together. And there are no words to thank someone who has taught you how to walk again.

That is why I never spoke the words to her…until now.

Iron sharpeneth iron; so a man sharpeneth the countenance of his friend.
~Proverbs 27:17

When The Student is Ready

Learning to stand was terrifying. To stand one must scoot to the edge of the chair, lean forward, and push still further forward while simultaneously rising up. Sounds easy? It's not. There is a split second in the mechanics of standing when you are looking downward still going in a forward momentum. For this split second of time, it seems as though you will topple forward to the floor.

As the therapist at Shepherd tried to talk me through the sequence of standing, she tried to convince me that my legs would not let me down. I began to breathe faster and I knew that a panic attack was not far away. How could I trust my legs, when my fingers did not perform on command, when my toes did not move when commanded? I had lost confidence in the ability of my brain to control functions in the other parts of my body. I was beginning to breathe fast, my heart pounded loudly in my chest, and I was beginning to panic. I was just too afraid to do it.

Finally, the therapist asked in a soothing voice, "Diane, maybe you should ask the doctor to give you something for anxiety?"

I looked at her and realized what she was saying. I needed yet another pill in my daily routine to make it through the day. I was already taking a paper cup full of pills at breakfast, lunch, and dinner. There were more pills before bedtime. I counted them one day and realized that I was taking almost thirty pills a day. Blood thinner, pain medication, and antibiotics were just a few in this endless list.

"Give me until tomorrow morning. If I still can't do this, I will ask him for something to help me."

When I had my talk with God that night, I asked him to help me conquer this fear. There was no clear answer, but I felt at peace. The next morning when we started again to go into the mechanics of standing I felt the anxiety starting to return. My therapist asked me if I could try to stand.

This was my answer. "I'll try." That hour I said only those two words whenever she asked me to do something. "I'll try" became my mantra. At the end of the hour I stood for the first time in months. And I didn't have to be medicated to face my fear! Today I stand and I don't even go through the mental sequence of how to do it. It has once again become an automatic action.

My next challenge would be relearning to walk. I was an outpatient at Pathways before I began to relearn the mechanics of walking. Fear edged back into my mind. At the end of the week I still fought that feeling of anxiety. When my driver dropped me off at home, I decided to stay on the front porch and enjoy the beautiful sunshine of a brilliant day.

Fall is a beautiful season. Camellia blooms of pink were translucent in the afternoon light, and the deep burgundy leaves of the weeping Japanese maple tree were stunning. I was admiring them and remembering when Scott and I had planted them so many years ago when I heard someone talking and looked toward our neighbor's house.

On Friday evenings our neighbors babysat their one-year-old grandson, Gabriel, whom they called Gabe.

He was learning to walk. He held his grandma's hands tightly, and wobbled trying to learn this new skill. Fascinated, I watched as he stretched out one foot, then the other, while clinging fearfully to grandma's hands. After successfully navigating a few steps, he lost his footing and stumbled. Grandma rescued him. After resting in Grandma's arms for a few moments, he struggled to get back down to the ground, and try again.

The following week in therapy, I pushed out the anxiety before it could put roots into my mind. If Gabe could face his fears and struggle to get back to the ground to try again, then so would I. I listened intently to my therapist. I asked her to let me walk in my walker more. Couldn't we do just one more lap? By the end of the week, I was using my walker exclusively in therapy.

The next Friday afternoon I once again sat on the porch. Gabe was now walking more sure-footed. He held on to one of his Grandma's hands. He was still walking flat-footed as all babies' start, but he was took time to enjoy this new trick he was learning. Every few steps he would stop and look around. He noticed everything, and looked as if he was getting great joy from this vertical way of viewing the world. Whenever a wondrous object caught his attention, he would walk over to it and inspect it closely. Then he would spy another wondrous thing, and walk nearer to examine it too. He was becoming a fearless walker.

That week in therapy, I moved in the walker with greater ease. I took time to appreciate the world from a vertical viewpoint. I began to walk fearlessly. I asked when I could use the walker at home. I was remembering the pure joy of taking a walk. Gabe was teaching me to rediscover the wonder of each new step in life.

On the third Friday night, I sat on the porch anxiously waiting to see Gabe. Finally, he and Grandma appeared in the driveway. He held her index finger and he was wearing brand new tennis shoes. He proudly extended his legs high in front of him as he walked, to better admire his new tennis shoes, reminding me of the magic P F Flyers in my own childhood. He was now completely comfortable on his feet and I knew that by next week he would be walking solo.

If I was to keep pace with Gabe, I needed more practice with the walker. The next afternoon, I set the brakes on my wheelchair and unfolded my walker. I began to walk down the hall toward the kitchen. As I passed my daughter's bedroom she opened her door to step out.

She squealed with delight, loudly announcing, "Mom, you are walking!" Both of my sons came rushing out of their rooms, and all three silently watched me walk into the kitchen.

Parents watch their children walk for the first time with great excitement. Few children get to experience this same joy as they watch their mother learn to walk again. We celebrated with hugs and tears.

Life is amazing and, oh so sweet!

When the student is ready the teacher will appear.
~ Zen Proverb

God's Timetable

There is a rhythm in healing that belongs only to God. It is like the gentle movement of the tide that methodically moves up the shore healing the sand of any blemishes. Just as the rhythm of the tide may vary in intensity, due to the external forces of the moon and weather, the rhythm of healing varies with the internal forces of attitude and faith.

Each day brought a challenge at Shepherd. For me it was not the challenge to overcome the pain that accompanies injuries and physical therapy, but the challenge to overcome fear that I fought the hardest. I experienced, and witnessed fear delay healing more than anything. Fear loomed in the darkest part of the mind, waiting for that toxic mixture of self-pity to unleash it to wreak havoc.

Mark Twain said, "Courage is resistance to fear, mastery of fear, not absence of fear."

At Pathways I learned to overcome fear best by watching those ahead of me. Their courage, determination, and words of praise allowed me to bask in soothing waves of healing. In turn, I helped others behind me find the strength to continue, to improve. Fear sometimes loomed large, but the rhythmic waves of healing that follow courage washed it away. All of this happened in God's perfect timetable.

I began to place greater trust in God, and as I looked for God's presence in my healing, I began to notice something else. Whenever something particularly disturbing or hard to overcome happened, an event would follow to cheer my spirit. I decided to think of these events as the thumbprints of God.

The day the audiologist told me I had severe hearing loss in both of my ears and would require hearing aids I returned to my room to find not one, but four cards from wonderful friends. Each card was filled with the perfect words of encouragement.

When the doctor at Emory Eye Clinic told me that my optic nerve had been irreparably damaged and I would never regain sight in my left eye, I tried hard to fight back tears. As I got into the van to go home, my driver handed me a package that had been given to him at Pathways. Inside the package I discovered a lovely crystal angel and a letter that told me, "You are up to this challenge!"

When I was told my right leg and foot might never improve, and I may never be able to wear two shoes, I expected a card or gift. On the long ride home I felt sure that God would once again make his presence known. I was disappointed to discover that I had not received any mail. Every other time I had received bad news, God had left a 'thumbprint' to let me know that he was with me and I could overcome this new obstacle. I had just decided to take a nap when the phone rang. It was the local florist asking for directions to my house. A friend had sent flowers. God was here!

When I tried to look too far into the future I became discouraged. I reminded myself that my timing is hurried and imperfect. I wanted to speed up my physical healing, but hadn't considered the mental and spiritual lessons tied to the holistic healing I was experiencing. I kept repeating to myself, "one day at a time." Then I saw the same message – "Take no thought for the morrow: for the morrow shall take thought for the things of itself. Sufficient unto the day is the evil thereof." Matthew 6:34

The challenges I will face today are enough. Looking ahead and trying to speed up the healing process will not work. God's timing is impeccable, sublime, and magnificent.

But I trusted in Thee O Lord: I said Thou art my God.
My times are in thy hands.
~ Psalms 31:14-15a

Insurance Questions

Of all of the experiences in this world called catastrophe, the worst for me was not the loss of mobility or brain function. My most dreaded experience was the inevitable process of dealing with insurance companies, and the bill collectors who don't care that this other entity is supposed to be paying. They have only one name – yours.

One of my conversations went something like this:

"Am I speaking to Mrs. Diane Quimby?"

"Yes, this is Diane Quimby."

"Mrs. Quimby, I need to talk with you about your claim. You did not provide complete information on original submission for coverage. This prevents us from paying the bill we have been receiving."

"When was the original paperwork submitted?"

"In November 2004," she replied. "Well, considering I was in a coma during that time I doubt I was able to provide much information."

"Well, Mrs. Quimby, it is more than just the original submission. There seems to be a discrepancy on your signature we need to discuss."

"Okay. What seems to be the problem with the signature?"

"Well your signature of February 2005 is markedly different from more recent signatures."

I thought a moment. "Let's see now" I replied. "In February 2005 my right hand was in a cast and I could not write with it. I am ruling out the option of writing holding the pen with my toes, because my toes didn't feel or move. There is the possibility that I wrote using my mouth, which might explain the sloppy nature of that signature. But I didn't have my top teeth implanted yet, so I probably couldn't have gummed the pen hard enough to sign the form you are talking about. I am going to venture a guess that since I only have one other hand that I wrote it with my left hand and that is why it is different."

"Really, Mrs. Quimby, there is no reason to be sarcastic. After all, I am just doing my job." She sounded rather nasty.

"I am not being sarcastic. I am trying to explore all possibilities of why my signature might be different. I want to dot all of the I's and cross all of the T's, because I don't want you to feel that you have left one single stone uncovered in resolving this matter. However, I am happy to hear of your diligence to your job. Perhaps you can explain why my doctor is going unpaid, why that past due bill is being turned over to collection agency, and why I keep getting all of these phone calls.

"Mrs. Quimby, if you have questions about this bill you will need to talk to someone in our customer service department."

"Great. Can you connect me with them please?"

"Certainly, who is your assigned to your file?"

"How should I know?" I answered testily.

"Well, your claim agent's name was listed on the form you received in December 2004."

"In December 2004 I had just come out of a coma and I don't remember specifically receiving or signing a form from your company.

"However, I did have a really remarkable hallucination while on medication about Godzilla. It wasn't the new Godzilla mind you, but the best Godzilla – the B movie Godzilla. I was sitting in the doctor's office and I looked out of the window to see thousands of doctors and nurses running down the hill screaming in terror. I was just deciding if I should start running too when Godzilla stepped right onto the entrance of the hospital crushing it to pieces. A really impressive hallucination, I still remember it so vividly. Now, let's get back to that form you were talking about…Hello…Hello?"

When at last we are sure you've been properly pilled,
then a few paper forms must be properly filled,
so that you and your heirs may be properly billed.
~Dr Seuss

The Miracle

When my catheter was removed, I was, at first, ecstatic. Later that night, when I could not tolerate even a single thimble full of urine in my bladder without feeling the desperate, urgent necessity of having to go to the bathroom, I was devastated. I rang for a tech to bring me a bedpan constantly throughout the night. It was the most degrading experience that I had yet endured. Being up all night dealing with this problem left me no courage or energy for therapy the next day.

General Patton said it best: "Fatigue makes cowards of us all."

As I sat in my wheelchair waiting for morning breakfast, I was no longer the woman I had known. I had mentally broken down, and I don't recall thinking anything. I began to silently cry. I don't know how long I sat there weeping, but soon I heard nurses and techs trying to talk to me. I had no energy for anyone, only a vague feeling of deep, inconsolable sadness. I remember someone giving me a shot before I was whisked back to my room and loaded back onto my bed.

Before I went to sleep, with a nurse's help, I called Scott. He had been to see me every night for weeks, and had planned to skip his visit this night, and go straight home for much needed rest.

When he answered, I told him, "Scott, I know you were planning to go home tonight, but I had a terrible night and day. I really need you." He assured me he would come. I hung up and fell asleep.

After lunch I went to afternoon therapy. I made progress in therapy and hoped that this would be enough to help me hang on through the night. Even though I really wanted him with me, I knew that Scott needed rest.

When I got back to my room, a tech helped me call, and I told him, "Don't come honey, I'm feeling better."

He said one sentence that meant everything; "I'm already on my way."

He entered my room without saying a word, and sat on the side of my bed. He put his arms around me, and for the first time since my horrible accident, I began to cry in grief.

I don't know how long I cried while he held me and stroked my hair, letting me get it all out. I do know that those tears were for everything I was experiencing; the loss of the person I had been, the loss of confidence, the loss of independence, and the growing realization that I might never regain the life I had always known. It felt heart wrenching, and strangely cleansing, to get these emotions out. Every hurt I had been feeling poured out of me like a fountain of grief that would not end until every drop was spent.

When I finally stopped crying, Scott talked with me. He told me that this was not the end of our story. He had big plans for us. He promised me that I would get better, and when I was better we were going on a cruise. He asked me where I would like to go. We planned a dream cruise that was far away from hospitals, and therapies, and everything that looked or sounded like the life we were currently enduring.

This promise of the cruise became the hope I worked toward. It took fourteen months, and I was still using a cane, when we boarded a Carnival Cruise ship bound for the Caribbean. Our neighbors went with us, and with much loving care from everyone, I had the time of my life.

On the first night of the cruise I could hear Scott's rhythmic breathing that told me he slept peacefully. I lay there thinking of all of the days that had led up to this cruise. I whispered a prayer of thanksgiving for life, for returning health, and for this man who had given so much to help me find my way back. I thought of my struggle to be free of the wheelchair, to regain thinking and reason, and the unlikely road that led me here, to this ship, sailing to islands I had only dreamed of seeing. Then I recalled the name of this ship and wondered why it had not jumped out at me immediately.

I smiled as I considered how very perfect it was that I was lying here beside a man I loved beyond measure. I looked through the glass door of my cabin onto a balcony suspended over the open seas of the Caribbean, visible by moonlight, on a ship called *The Miracle*.

The world is round and the place which may seem like the end may also be only the beginning
~ Ivy Baker Priest

Miserable Comforters

Job called them miserable comforters, and you have met them too. They are the ones who come to bring comfort and leave ruin and despair in their wake. The young doctor at Memorial University Medical Center who felt it was his duty to seek out my husband to tell him that I would not live – a miserable comforter. The nurse, who sees her position as a point of power, and long ago lost the fire of comforting the sick, is a miserable comforter. The friend who comes under the guise of bringing words of solace, but leaves you feeling despair or anger at their complete lack of understanding in matters of faith, hope, or common courtesy – a miserable comforter.

I met Michael, a husband of thirty years, married to a woman who had sustained a traumatic brain injury. His wife did not yet remember him and he could finally say this out loud without breaking down into tears. A "good friend" had just come to visit. In one brief visit full of thoughtless comments, this friend left with Michael's wife so distraught that it took medication and hours to calm her – another miserable comforter.

Anyone who has spent any time in a hospital has encountered a miserable comforter. It is important to understand how to protect your loved one and yourself from these negative influences. You know that you are having a "Job" moment when a hospital visit starts off positive and ends with a negative statement causing you to question your own positive outcome.

Miserable comforters arrive when you are in crisis and visit with every intention of comforting you. They say things like, "I have a friend who had cancer, too. Bless her heart she really suffered before she finally died. Come to think of it, her cancer was not as far along as yours."

Whatever your malady, they appear like crows circling a cornfield. However, if you expect them and guard your heart, you can maintain a straighter path to healing. A caregiver of one TBI survivor confided that she strictly limited her husband's visitors early on. He had already had too many incidents of miserable comforters to allow his well-being to be sidetracked.

How can you guard against a miserable comforter? Here's how Job handled the situation. "Then Job answered and said, 'I have heard many such things: miserable comforters are ye all. Shall vain words have an end? Or what emboldeneth thee that thou answerest? I could also speak as ye do; if your soul were in my soul's stead, I could heap up words against you and shake mine head at you. But I would strengthen you with my mouth, and the moving of my lips should assuage your grief.'" Job 16:1-5

My personal version is: "You are all miserable comforters. Can't you just keep your mouth shut? Do you always have to have the last word? I could speak like you if you were in my place. I could say hurtful, thoughtless words and shake my head at you, but I would rather seek to strengthen you with kind words to lessen your pain."

It is usually the miserable comforter who leaves the hospital visit oblivious to the pain they have caused, and it is the patient who is frazzled at the end of the visit. But this is not always the case. A good friend told me about a miserable comforter visit that had the reverse effect.

Her husband was in the very early days of his TBI. It is not unusual for a patient during this time to use extensive profanity. TBI survivors who never used profanity before their injury may briefly cuss like sailors. Her husband was one of them. These TBI survivors are surprised and embarrassed when they learn of this later, because they have no memory of this event.

She and her children were so delighted that he was finally speaking they didn't care what he said. Her husband's brother came with a fellow church member for a visit. Each time her husband uttered a profanity, this pious gentleman would stop him in what he was saying and lecture him. My friend had just decided to cut this visit, and the profanity lectures, short when her husband let loose with a string of profane sentences using every profane word she had ever heard and had even included a few newly made up words to go along with them.

When he finished ranting, there was silence. The church friend and brother decided to leave and offered to pray before leaving. The brother prayed lifting her husband's injuries to God. When the pious friend prayed, he asked God to remove the profanity from her husband. There was no prayer for healing, and no prayer for comfort for the family, only that her husband would quit using profanity.

When he finished praying the visitor looked solemnly at her husband and said, "Now, can you remember what I prayed? Can you remember not to use profanity?"

Her husband, in complete innocence, responded, "I'll try, but it's so fucking hard."

Never let your sense of morals get in the way of doing what is right. ~ Isaac Asimov

Oh, Well...

All of us handle traumatic brain injury in our own way. Occasionally, someone really captures the essence of how it feels. David was one guy who summed it up perfectly. He would exhale a deep sigh and then say, to no one in particular, "Oh well, what the hell. Watcha gonna do?" Only he didn't rush the words. He put a pause in after every couple of words to give proper emphasis to his predicament. It sounded more like an extension of his sigh than words. He repeated this one sentence over and over and over. He said this frequently throughout the day. In fact, he said it so often that one table of patients had a running bet going on how long it would take before he said it after joining them at the table for breakfast each day.

I met David and his parents while peer visiting. He looked to be in his mid-twenties and was in a wheelchair. A car had run a stop sign, and he had hit it broadside with his motorcycle. He had been wearing a helmet and his prognosis was good.

He knew that with hard work and determination he would one day walk again. David and his parents were from Ohio. His parents had traveled to Atlanta to be with him and were staying in an apartment provided for family members. Both were immaculately dressed and had impeccable manners. During our first visit, he kept repeating his favorite phrase and I could see his mother flinch involuntarily each time he said it. From her conservative dress and temperament, I felt sure that David's motto was straining her nerves, but she never let on. There was just the involuntary flinch in her face each time he said it.

On our next visit David had decided to stay in his room and rest. As we talked I noticed that this impeccably dressed mom and dad were starting to show the strain of their second week of coping with David's traumatic brain injury. I reminded them that they needed to take care of themselves. His mother quickly assured me that they were getting rest. We talked about David's improvements and discussed his upcoming transfer. Finally, we discussed the eventual care giving that David would require at home. I listened as his mother listed options and her nervousness at her ability to handle all of David's needs.

Before I even had a chance to provide additional resources she said almost wistfully and without the slightest hint of a flinch, "Oh well, what the hell. Watcha gonna do?"

Another patient voiced the essence of his brain injury by frequently repeating one sentence. He was a huge, burly construction worker. His therapist smiled as she remembered his standard reply when he was asked how he was doing.

He solemnly answered, "I'm too lovely for this."

To this statement I heartily agree. Traumatic brain injury is called the silent epidemic with good reason. Each of us struggles to find our voice. It may be a silent voice, or it may sound like guttural grunts, it could be a voice temporarily laced with profanity, but it is the collective and lovely voice of a brain-injured community refusing to give up.

For all of us – all one million seven hundred thousand newly brain-injured people in the U.S. each year, and for the thousands who go undiagnosed, we may begin with the anthem, "Oh well, what the hell. Watcha gonna do?" but we are moving on with post it notes, calendars, endless lists, and small notebooks to record information we may forget, because we are too lovely for this.

We may have all come on different ships,
but we're in the same boat now.
~ Martin Luther King, Jr.

Primordial Instinct

In my last month of outpatient therapy I saw Dylan for the first time. He had been in the car with three other teenagers. He was sat in the back seat and his younger sister had been in the front. The driver, his sister, and another passenger had all been killed in the collision. Dylan lived. I use the term lived to mean that he still breathed, because there was very little else to call a life remaining. Being in the midst of catastrophe for eleven months can make you tough, but this sight brought me to tears.

Dylan's accident had happened two years earlier. His body had drawn up with his arms and legs unable to extend fully. His shell of a body was housed in a wheelchair and his head drooped to the left. His eyes focused straight ahead – on nothing. No one knew if he could still see, or process what he saw. He could hear, but he could not speak. His mother and father hoped that therapy would help him regain some mobility in his limbs. With each touch by the therapist he would cry out, like a baby with a very low voice. Only his mother's patient uttering in his ear could calm him.

I consider it a miracle that on my final day as an outpatient, Dylan was also there, and I could see improvement in him. His parents suffering through the loss of their only daughter now dedicated themselves to caring for their remaining child.

I remember the joy I felt when I held each of my children for the first time. I don't think any parent holds their newborn baby, and sees this picture as a possible future for their child. Dylan's parents were extraordinary people. With no outside help other than therapy, and with no response or acknowledgement from their son, they were committed to give him the best life available. They were patient and loving. I think of them both when I see selfish or self-centered attitudes in others, and I am guided to be a better person.

I feel inadequate to describe this amazing love and commitment I have seen in the parents of TBI survivors. Within seconds of hearing there is an emergency involving their child, parents leave their homes and jobs, and everything is suspended to be near the child. All plans, all appointments, all commitments have ceased to exist. There is only one agenda – their child. The universe is aligned for visiting hour, and the telephone to send out the latest news. There is no hunger, no sleep – only prayer and hope, hope and prayer. Yesterday's routine is shattered and all thought is directed to the latest update from the doctor. Life is described in percentages, and medical procedures are described in cautionary words that won't give, and yet, won't deny hope. It is a roller coaster ride with no certain end.

I have come to believe that a primordial instinct lies dormant in the heart of a parent, because I have seen it awakened. This instinct remains unseen in the everyday world, but in crisis it becomes the raw power of love unleashed. This is the instinct that we see sometimes in animals when their babies are threatened. It is a sparrow who flies recklessly after a hawk, chasing it from the skies, away from her nest; a loving pet who growls and bares her teeth when you approach her nursing pups. It is magnificent to behold. I have seen this same instinct unveil in parents of TBI survivors. I am humbled by their love and devotion.

When I held my oldest son, Anthony, for the first time, I experienced a love that I did not know existed. I was filled with selfless unconditional love that placed his needs firmly above mine. I imagine that this love I have seen in TBI parents comes from the same place. It never ceases to to fill me with awe. I have met so many of these parents, and I have finally learned the important lesson that all of them have taught me. Don't put it off until later. No one ever regrets the love given to his or her child. Show your child this magnificent love that comes from a place they do not even know exists.

Don't wait. Say it now. Do it now.

While we try to teach our children all about life,
our children teach us what life is all about.
~ Angela Schwindt

Dress Shoes

My answering machine delivered the news that Dr. Brenda Watts Jones, a woman I greatly admired, had died of inflammatory breast cancer. I stood glued to the floor in disbelief. She was only a year older than me. She had a son still in school. Her husband and family were surely devastated that a life so full of energy and drive had been so suddenly extinguished.

Dr. Jones greatly influenced my life. I regret that I never took the time to tell her that I considered her the epitome of a brilliant professional. She came to Atlanta Technical College as its fifth president of the college since I had been employed as a carpentry instructor. I was amazed at how she had improved the school. She was strictly business. I would never have felt comfortable calling her anything but Dr. Jones. She wanted all staff to be appropriately dressed at all times. She expected nothing less than your best effort. It had been nine years since I had worked at Atlanta Tech, but I still considered myself a part of that family. As I prepared to go the memorial service in Dr. Jones's honor, I considered what shoes to wear.

My husband had once called me Imelda Marcos. My love of shoes had not rivaled her 1,000 plus collection, but my feet certainly knew how to style. Since the wreck, I had searched in vain for regular shoes that would fit my swollen right foot. At this time I owned only a pair of men's tennis shoes and a pair of black orthopedic dress shoes that I felt sure I would not be able to get onto my right foot.

In the struggle with a traumatic brain injury, it seems sometimes bizarre how we deal with the loss of the former self. My inability to walk sure-footedly sometimes paled in comparison to my desire to once again wear attractive shoes. I think this desire said less about wanting great looking shoes, and more about the desire to be who I once was. This greater understanding and acceptance had not yet come, and at the time I saw it only as a shoe problem.

The thought of what Dr. Jones would think if she saw me in tennis shoes at her memorial service left me no choice. I pulled out the black shoes and stuffed my right foot in. The response was immediate – pain! Since I had been able to get the shoe on, I wasn't about to take it off. As I drove to the memorial service, I felt Dr. Jones's eyes on me. I pictured her as I drove, shaking her head and saying to herself, "Tennis shoes at my memorial service? Girl, I can't believe you even considered it." This thought made me laugh.

It felt good to see so many old friends, even if we were there for a very sad reason. As the service began, my foot ached and continued to swell. Eventually, I began to think the sides of the shoe would burst open. Then, even later, I began to hope it would, but it didn't. That black dress shoe stayed together. Knowing Dr. Jones's take charge spirit, it wouldn't surprise me, some day when I join her, to learn that she assigned angels to keep that shoe from splitting apart.

There are many things that we regret in life. Not telling Dr. Jones what an outstanding person I thought she was is one of mine. I would like to think that wearing those dress shoes was my way of showing my respect to her, my own personal expression of how I valued her influence on me. But if I'm really honest with myself, there was another reason even more important. I will admit that even in death this woman held me to her high standards. I don't want our first meeting in Eternity to begin by explaining why I wore men's tennis shoes to her memorial service.

It is only when we truly know and understand that we have a limited time on earth – and that we have no way of knowing when our time is up – that we will begin to live each day to the fullest, as if it was the only one we had. ~ Elisabeth Kubler-Ross

The Rock and the Stream

While still struggling to master the use of a cane, I attended group therapy sessions with people who looked whole. Mark, a fellow patient, once told me that I was *lucky* to have so many medical problems and injuries, because people could look at me and believe that I had sustained a traumatic brain injury. Since that time, I have even encountered doctors who do not understand traumatic brain injury. I sustained a fracture to my skull, was blinded in my left eye, crushed my left sinus cavity, fractured the bones in my upper mouth creating a gaping wound in the top of my mouth, knocked out every tooth in my upper mouth except one, sustained severe hearing loss required hearing aids, and paralysis on one side of my face.

These are verifiable injuries that occurred to my head, but to consider that this impact has also impaired my brain's capabilities remains incomprehensible for some doctors. If some in the medical profession still don't understand traumatic brain injury, how can an employer, a spouse and family, a friend, an insurance adjuster, or a judge presiding at a disability hearing grasp this truth? The common rule seems to be that if the brain injury is not severe enough to cause inability to speak or perform the most basic of functions, then it cannot be real. A frustrating and sad truth begins to dawn on me. Under the current medical and legal system, I could actually receive greater help for an impaired finger or toe, than for my impaired brain. That is the bizarre reality that Mark was talking about so many years ago.

The numbers game that is played by insurance providers works against those who have survived TBI. The unwritten motto seems to be a cleverly jumbled version of the old adage, "out of sight, out of mind" distorted into "out of mind, out of sight." Since the insurance adjusters cannot see this injury, it does not exist. TBI survivors in the extreme categories are acknowledged, and in most cases treatment is approved. However, I have seen survivors even in this category initially refused coverage. TBI survivors in the mild to moderate range face an uphill battle.

A friend recounted a story that her son told her. Her son, a Marine, was stationed in Hawaii. As he left the PX one day, he encountered another young Marine standing outside in tears. He stopped and asked this young man if he could help. The soldier, recently stateside from Iraq, told him that he had been in a vehicle that had been blasted apart by a roadside bomb. Since that time, he'd had trouble remembering events, and performing his job. His sergeant had just informed him that he would receive a dishonorable discharge if he continued to perform his duties in such a haphazard way. Having grown up with a dad who had survived a TBI, my friend's son recognized immediately that this soldier had an undiagnosed TBI. I can only hope that this soldier received the help he needed.

Early rehabilitative treatment for TBI, ensures the best results. The numbers game played by insurance companies is betting that if they deny the original claim, you will give up and go away. I cannot stress how important it is to keep fighting for yourself, or for your loved one. Do some research and retain a lawyer to advocate for you. An attorney can fight for your rights, and will not bill you unless you receive compensation. You *must* be persistent.

The system is set up to discourage people, and many do give up. Social Security routinely denies claims in hopes that the injured person will just go away. Appeal these decisions! I know of cases that should have been approved immediately and were denied *three or more times* before the TBI survivor was approved for compensation. TBI rehabilitation is critical and the fight may be long, but living with a TBI without rehabilitation is to doom yourself or your loved one to a substandard life.

At the moment of your injury, your life and all of your hopes and dreams became a game of percentages. Your opponent in this game knows the rules. Your opponent hopes that if you appeal and are denied, you will give up the fight. Many survivors or family members do give up and the actual cost to the insurance provider becomes less each time. Don't give up! You may be denied two, three, or even four times, and this circuitous process will not stop until you retain an attorney.

I lived in limbo for three and a half years before I received a semi-resolution and still have outstanding issues. I have learned one truth in this matter – you do not know the rules of this game. An attorney does. Retain a good attorney, one specializing in your specific needs and specific insurance area, and you have an excellent chance of receiving the financial help you need to pay for the services necessary to reclaim your life. Continue to fight for your benefits, and seek your day in court if necessary. Don't become an insignificant number. Our struggles are unique. We are not claim numbers. We are an integral part of this silent epidemic. We need to stop being so silent.

The causes of a TBI are countless: a car accident, a diving accident, a motorcycle accident, a bike wreck, a brain tumor, a stroke, a war casualty, a simple fall. In other words, anyone could join our ranks. If we are to make the path easier for those who will travel behind us, we must continue to advocate for for ourselves and others. Only then can we break the cloak of silence that renders us invisible.

In the confrontation between the stream and the rock, the stream always wins – not through strength but by perseverance. ~ H. Jackson Brown, Jr.

All the King's Horses

I live the land of halfway. No longer bound to a wheelchair, I do not yet have the steady, balanced walk of my past. It has taken me longer than most of peers, but I am finally here. This last leg of the journey is not the most painful, but it is the most frustrating. I can almost see the light at the end of the tunnel.

The right foot I'd hoped would regain sensation has severed nerves that will not repair. The swelling in the foot and leg has not subsided, a permanent casualty of the accident. My facial paralysis remains. Many years and more surgeries than I can count, I am finally looking at the home stretch. A final operation looms in the future. I tell myself, "Just one more year."

Like the tortoise in the immortal race, slow and steady, that's me. In my low times, I compare myself to Humpty Dumpty, learning that there are some things that simply cannot be put back together again. In my good times, I shake off what is lost and no longer yearn for things that were. I am thankful for things that remain.

Yet, in my dreams, I am always whole. I sometimes wonder, as more time passes if I will begin to dream of myself as I am now. In those dreams, will I become the woman who can't think of words, can't remember complete thoughts, who is easily distracted? Or will my innermost self always see the woman I was?

I begin to understand why patients in the spinal cord injury unit are thankful not to be in the acquired brain injury (ABI) unit. Consider life in a wheelchair with a functioning brain vs. walking with a dysfunctional brain. What would be your choice? Since none of us are given the opportunity to choose, we must make the most of what we have. I will say that I have learned to accept my physical limitations much easier than my mental ones. Being unable to walk for almost a year was not nearly as frustrating as trying to remember where I lived, what my house looks like, remembering my family, remembering how to get to places where I have been often, or losing the ability to easily track sentences when I read.

My brain injury allows me to remember how I was before the wreck, while understanding better with each passing day of how different I am now. I have yet to figure out how to resolve this conundrum. Experientially, my brain says it will take me thirty minutes to pay the bills. For thirty years this has been the case. Today, it is up in the air. Some days it takes an hour, and other days it takes two.

This fine line between faith and denial is easily crossed and one person's faith may be another person's denial. An early counselor talked about the five stages of grief: denial, anger, bargaining, depression, and acceptance. Where am I today? Where is anyone for that matter? Unless we have faced no adversity at all, then all of us are in one of the five stages. Divorce, natural disasters, disease, accidents, betrayal of trust from someone close, the death of a loved one, estrangement from a family member, the list is endless. To dwell on these dark times and never think of the periods of light can take one on a fast spiral down. Is the glass half full or half empty? Will you get better or get bitter?

My personal armor as I journey through these dark times has been my deepening spiritual awareness. My belief is that people and circumstances are never perfect and will sometimes let me down. It is my unshakable faith that God will never let me down that keeps me going. God has become my resting place. I pray that you will find yours.

Mishaps are like knives, that either serve us or cut us,
as we grasp them by the blade or the handle.
~ James Russell Lowell

A Friend in Deed

Within tragedy are hidden moments, like gold nuggets, that beg to be noticed. Sometimes we get so caught up in the tragedy that we don't notice these moments that lie there, waiting to be plucked up to offer us hope in this sea of sorrow. Good friends keep us anchored in this raging sea.

My main anchor was Diane Reeves. During those first days after the wreck, she went to Savannah. My family had been camped out in the waiting room for several days when she showed up with a cooler of delicious homemade pound cake, banana nut bread, sandwiches, and drinks. She came with everything my family needed to be comfortable. She listened. She encouraged. She was perfect.

The night before I was transferred to Shepherd, she was there. I have a brief flash of memory of her feeding me Jello. She was at Shepherd frequently. She brought me sweat suits, washed my clothes, applied lotion, performed a vinegar treatment to my hands and arms to remove scaly dried out skin. She arranged my room, checked my schedule and my progress frequently. When I transferred to Pathways, she came and packed my things. She arranged my new room, and then stayed to have lunch with me to help me fit in with the new routine. She was, and is, the perfect friend. I can never repay her for her love and care.

Anne Welch was another great friend. She called me frequently at Pathways. She always had a humorous story or the perfect words to lift me up. She was great support and kept me moving toward independence.

Patti Fields took on a project to make a quilt for me, never dreaming it would become so time consuming. She was another light in the darkness.

My two Susan's (Brown and Evans) from work sent me a care basket of wonderful spa treatments.

Rueben Guilliame was a frequent visitor in Savannah, and later at Shepherd. Rueben was there to direct Scott to my new room when I was moved out of the MST ward in Savannah.

There are so many people who have given so much. It was tempting to overlook this love and concentrate instead on the loss. Fortunately, I recognized these golden moments and great thankfulness grew in my heart leaving no room for bitterness to grow.

Isn't this the essence of good friends? They carry you when you can't carry yourself. They bring light when it is dark. They give you the pat on the back or the swift kick in the pants when needed. They are the people you choose to journey beside through life. They are the cream that rises to the top when tragedy churns the milk. They are the essential ingredients in a life worth living. They are love in deeds.

If you have a true friend, then you have more than your share. ~ Thomas Fuller

Ramona

She is the gentle reminder of how wondrous it feels to be unconditionally loved. A simple trip to the grocery store and she acts like I have been gone for weeks. Animals are wonderful companions, and she is the most wonderful of all.

I had too much alone time on my hands. I asked Scott if he minded if we went to the pound and got a puppy. He agreed and on the following day Kelly, Anthony, and I went to pick out a puppy. I gazed into one cage to find three black and white puppies from the same litter. Two of the puppies were at the front of the cage wagging their tails and I felt sure they would find a nice home. One puppy was in the back corner of the cage and did not move. She looked afraid and vulnerable. I picked her.

On the way out of the puppy area we passed grown cats in cages. One cat extended her paw as if saying, "Take me too!" My daughter pleaded to get her and when I said yes, she gave her brother a thumbs up.

When we got home we started trying out names on the new cat and puppy. Kelly promptly named the cat Dagny. I named the puppy Ramona. Within hours Ramona got sick. I rushed her to the vet and arrived just before closing on that Friday afternoon. He checked her for parvo, a disease that I had never heard of, and told me that the results were negative. He told me that there could be any number of reasons for her to be queasy, but that she should be fine.

Only she wasn't. On Saturday morning, she became even sicker and weaker. I watched over her carefully. Late on Sunday night she began to foam at the mouth. I quickly woke my daughter. She drove us to an all-night pet emergency room thirty minutes away. They tested Ramona again for parvo and this time the results came back positive. I learned that parvo is a viral killer of puppies. Parvovirus has a 50% mortality rate. She was hooked up to an IV. When they released her I was instructed to take her to the vet for additional treatment.

We took her back to the vet as soon as he opened that morning and she became an animal hospital patient for ten days. I visited her every morning and every afternoon. I watched helplessly as she continued to decline. My once pretty little puppy had become an emaciated, sad looking animal. Each visit saw no improvement, but I continued to visit and to hold her wrapped in a blanket talking soothingly to her and telling her how much I wanted her to come home. On the fifth day I began to wonder if I should allow this poor animal to continue to suffer. How much longer should she suffer before I told the vet to end her suffering?

On Sunday, Scott went with me to visit Ramona. She could no longer sit or stand. I held her wrapped in a blanket and prayed silently. I thanked God for allowing me to be a friend to Ramona. I told him that I could finally let her go, and take the lesson that my part in our friendship had been to bring comfort to a sick puppy in her short time of life, if that was what my role was to be. As we drove home Scott was unusually quiet. I asked if he thought Ramona would live. He smiled a weak smile and said nothing. Each time I thought of her that night I whispered a little prayer for her.

On Monday morning I went to the vet's office to visit Ramona in the infirmary and found an assistant cleaning her cage. I couldn't see her so I asked anxiously, "How is she?" The assistant slowly shook her head. When she moved out of the way I opened the door and began to talk to Ramona. Slowly, with excruciating effort, she sat up. Her legs trembled with the effort, but she was sitting. I knew that challenge of sitting up again after an endless time of lying. I quickly grabbed a blanket and held her, praising her for her extraordinary effort. Each day thereafter I saw improvement. Finally, she was able to once again walk and she could come home. She was weak and emaciated, but improving.

That is how Ramona Quimby got her start in our family and into my heart. She is the doggie version of an ultimate survivor spirit. She is my loyal companion. Through all of my surgeries she has been a steadfast friend. After my most recent surgery, she laid on the bed with me and refused to leave. Kacy had to carry her outside to go to the bathroom. Then she immediately returned to my room to keep her silent vigil with me.

I could have chosen any puppy at the pound. There was something about Ramona that called out to me. She is not a handsome dog. She has mismatched, lopsided ears, and a wonderful eclectic array of black and white toenails. She is a medium sized dog. There is nothing physically striking about her. Most people would see nothing special at all.

Unconditional, loving loyalty, and steadfast friendship are only visible to the heart.

Dogs are not our whole life, but they can make our lives whole. ~ Roger Caras

Amerigo Vespucci

Each year 1.7 million Americans sustain a traumatic brain injury. 80,000 people will experience a long-term disability due to the injury, and 52,000 Americans will not survive a traumatic brain injury.[1] Every 23 seconds someone in the U.S. sustains a traumatic brain injury. An estimated 3.1 million Americans currently live with disabilities resulting from traumatic brain injury.[2]

Sometimes I imagine all of us as a computer generated collage picture of a brain. Zoom in on this picture and view the individual photos of each of us who make up the whole picture and read our unique stories. These stories are composites of strength and weakness, faith and fear, celebration and depression that simultaneously mourn the death of the old life, and exalt in determination to find the new life. We all aspire to walk, to dress ourselves, to talk, to swallow, to eat, to think, to control our emotions, to regain the dignity and self-respect we once took for granted. It is the yin and yang of the journey from tragic loss to glorious

[1] Cited from statistics on the Center for Disease Control (CDC) 2012 website (www.cdc.gov/traumaticbraininjury/tbi_ed.html)
[2] Cited from statistics on the Brain Injury Association of America (BIAA) 2012 website (www.biausa.org/)

independence and all of the detours and side roads that must be traveled along this road to healing.

We all begin our journey in this new world of confusion and we must learn to navigate our own way. There is no one-size-fits-all map that directs us onto the path of independence. We must find it on our own, if that option is available to us. Many others have traveled a similar path and they can help us find places of solace in this journey. Support groups are one place of solace. It is there that we discover that we are not alone. Many of our feelings are common feelings shared by all of us. Information and advice is available there, friends for both the survivor and the caregiver are found there.

Counseling is another place of solace. A professional counselor with thorough knowledge of traumatic brain injury can be a critical guide in navigating these new paths. Strategies for success are shared and we come faster to a new life of independence with the help of a competent counselor. I have met many capable people who sustained their brain injury over ten years ago living very fulfilling lives. I have met few who have achieved this level of success without participation in a support group, private counseling, or therapy somewhere along the way.

It is so easy to become reclusive. If we don't leave the house, we don't have to find our way in the new world around us. It can be a cause of stress and anxiety to interact with impatient people who won't spare the extra few seconds to explain a confusing procedure or policy. But we must persist. We are now in a new and uncharted territory. If we want to provide others coming behind us with a better map of how to travel this terrain we must become fearless navigators in our personal journey.

America is named for Amerigo Vespucci, an Italian navigator and explorer. It was he who determined that Columbus and others were not sailing to China, but to an uncharted territory of a new world. I have met the Amerigo Vespucci for traumatic brain injury in Georgia. Her name is Ann Boriskie, and she is the creator and administrator of the Peer Visitor Program for traumatic brain injury in Georgia.

She facilitates training for other survivors of TBI, and she coordinates this program of TBI survivors and caregivers who volunteer among the many hospitals and the veterans' administration in the metro Atlanta area. She has written a business plan for the program and secures funding for this program. She pays many of the administrative expenses for this program out of her own pocket. What she has accomplished is incredible. Her understanding of the needs of TBI survivors and caregivers is thorough and extensive. Through her efforts and the efforts of other TBI volunteers, thousands of TBI survivors and their families have been given critical information and support when they need it most. When you consider that she is also a TBI survivor, her accomplishments are even more remarkable.

Each of us has the potential to be an incredibly positive influence on others if we take just one moment to reach back and help someone behind move a little farther along the path.

You will rise by lifting others. ~ Robert Green Ingersoll

A Fleeting Thought

A fleeting thought, like a puff of smoke released into the air, it vanishes before it can be captured. Like Sisyphus eternally rolling a rock up a mountain only to watch it roll back down. That is how it is.

I am thirsty. I go to the kitchen. I see that the trash needs to be emptied. I empty the trashcan and replace the bag. I wipe down the counter top and load a few dishes into the dishwasher. I return to my computer and sit down. Then I remember that I am thirsty.

I go into the kitchen and see the bills lying on the kitchen desk. I decide to pay the bills. But first I must find my pocketbook with my calculator inside. I find my pocketbook and while walking through the office I see that my computer is on and I sit down. Then I remember that I am thirsty.

I go to the kitchen and again see the bills on the desk. I remember that I was going to pay the bills. I go back into my bedroom to find my pocketbook. It is not there. I begin to panic. Where did I put my pocketbook? Where did I have it last? Did I leave it in the van? I go to the van and look, but it is not there. I try to remember where I was yesterday that I might have left my pocketbook. I search and search. I become frustrated. Finally, I decide to go to my office and work on my computer. There is my pocketbook. Why was I looking for my pocketbook? I can't remember. So I sit down at my computer and then I remember that I am thirsty.

The world of traumatic brain injury is a fleeting thought. Like a puff of smoke that is released into the air, it vanishes before it can be captured. Like Sisyphus eternally rolling a rock up a mountain only to watch it roll back down.

That is how it is.

We are made to persist. That's how we find out who we are. ~ Tobias Wolff

All I Know of Angels

It was Christmas time at Shepherd Center and my sister-in-law, Denise, had a surprise for me. She had been in contact with hundreds of my friends and professional associates and had created a beautiful angel tree. It was over six feet tall, and was a spiral of lights growing ever larger to the floor. It had beautiful angel ornaments wound throughout. Doctor Bilsky had come into my room and proclaimed it the most beautiful Christmas tree at Shepherd. Denise also presented me with a huge book. On each page was a large photo of each individual ornament with the accompanying card from the giver. It was a magnificent gift of love and my most memorable Christmas gift ever.

She and Doug traveled from Tennessee to set the tree up for me and she had personally packed each ornament when it was taken down so that no harm came to any ornament. After I came home the question became what to do with all of these lovely angel ornaments? I decided to display them on shelves in my living room every day of the year. As I walk through the living room each day I see them all and I think of the people who prayed for me, and I feel incredibly blessed.

The daily sight of this multitude of angel ornaments led me to become curious and to do some biblical research on angels. The first thing I learned is that there is no written account of angels having wings in the Bible. In fact, it is quite the opposite. Most often angels were mistaken for people. I imagine that a huge pair of wings mounted on someone's back would definitely rule out mistaking them for human.

One other thing I noticed is that there is no account in the Bible of a female angel. All accounts of an angel in the Bible either specifically mention a male or don't specify any gender. I am not saying they don't exist, only that there is no written account of a woman angel.

I learned that angels are celestial beings that have specific orders. They have been sent as messengers from God telling us things we need to know. They have been sent to fight for us in the spiritual realm we don't see. Everyone has heard the term guardian angel, and I think the angel at Memorial University Medical Center sat there to protect and guard over me.

Although my understanding of celestial angels may be limited, my knowledge of people who bring the comfort of an angel is extensive. Denise was an angel. She kept a prayer email chain for me and sent daily medical reports of what was happening to everyone who knew me, encouraging those on the list to forward to others. This email report was distributed to hundreds of people. They became my prayer warriors. She tells me that she witnessed miracles early in my treatment. One miracle occurred when the doctor told my family that they needed to amputate my right leg. She led a prayer, as they took me into surgery. During the surgery one of the doctors had a flash of inspiration to try an unusual procedure before performing the amputation. I returned from surgery with two legs.

Later, when I was at Shepherd, I only had to mention I needed or wanted something and Doug and Denise would provide it. A slice of watermelon in mid-

December? No problem. Reading glasses? No problem. Their love for me ensured that I had anything I wanted or needed. How can I ever thank them for such love? Isn't this the common trait that we associate with celestial angels? They offer such comfort, such care that no thanks offered that can match their gift. So God, the great Giver of Love, receives the praise.

My friends in the National Association of Women in Construction (NAWIC) were great angels of comfort to me. They mounted a card campaign to encourage me. When I first began to understand and remember things, my family told me they would bring in some of the cards that had been sent to me. I never expected two large boxes of cards. I cannot express how these wonderful women touched me in this gesture. There were hundreds of cards from women all over the country. Many of these cards were from people I didn't even know. They were powerful encouragement and offered the light of love in a dark time.

My Region 2 NAWIC friends created a lovely quilt that contained messages of love, hope, encouragement, and scriptures. It hangs on my wall in the hallway of my home to remind me not to get discouraged. Women from Alabama, Georgia, and Tennessee traveled to surprise me. I was living at Pathways. My husband and children were there when they surprised me with this amazing gift. I cried so hard at this gesture of love. When I looked up they were crying, too. It was not the small cry of few tears, but the sobs of joy unleashed. Real joy is like that; it gives tears to express what the heart cannot utter into words.

My friends from work at BE&K, Inc. were also angels of love. On the day following my wreck, the company's Chairman of the Board and the CEO sent an email throughout the building informing all employees that at 11:00 that morning any employee who wanted to pray on my behalf could gather at the flagpole in front of the building to pray for me. Promptly at 11:00, the entire building emptied. 600 people gathered and prayed for me. I attribute my survival directly to this concentrated prayer. Employees also took up a collection for my family for Christmas. A $1,200 gift card was given to Scott and the kids to purchase gifts. This extraordinary gesture is reminiscent of the Frank Capra movie, *It's a Wonderful Life*. This great outpouring of love is beyond my ability to describe.

The final lesson I learned in my research about angels is that in many conversations recorded of an angel speaking with a person, the angel begins the conversation with two words: Fear not. Fear can hinder, fear can shut down the mind, and, if we let it, fear can defeat us. Fear is the great bluff. It stands between our dreams and us. In reality, it is a barrier of nothing, that we sometimes give power over everything. Fear was my enemy in relearning to walk. I realized that fear has always been my enemy in every area of my life when I stepped out and tried something new or significant. I have learned that when I get too comfortable, I am not growing. It is only in the discomfort of reaching out to a new goal that I face the fear inherent in taking on a new challenge. I've learned to trust the angels on this one.

Fear not.

Be not forgetful to entertain strangers; for thereby some have entertained angels unawares. ~ Hebrews 13: 2

No Excuses

I was walking toward the peer visiting room when I ran into a therapist who had been instrumental in helping me in my early struggles. She and I were reminiscing about my time at Shepherd. Although I don't remember those first days of anger, I was not surprised when she told me that she was one of the people I had fired on my first day. Another therapist approached us while we were talking and told me that I had fired her every day for a week. I think she holds the current record, although I won't rule out the possibility that someday someone else will tell me that I fired him or her even more. If that ever happens, it won't come as a surprise to me. However, one thing I learned in our conversation did surprise me.

As we talked, my therapist told me that my husband had been standing beside my bed when I was firing everyone. I felt stunned. In all of this time he has never mentioned to me that he was there. I thought about this and considered all of the completely off-the-wall, bizarre, even crazy moments he has witnessed since I sustained my injury. Never one time in all of these years has he brought up anything I did or said. I think of this and become even more convinced that the greatest preparation anyone can have, to face catastrophe, is supportive love from family and friends, and a strong spiritual base. With these two foundations, any tragedy becomes easier to bear.

I cannot express how vital it was for me to have Scott with me. I don't believe words were ever intended to convey the depths of a person's heart. That is the purpose of tears, and warm, encompassing hugs. Sometimes I am overwhelmed with love and gratitude for this gift of someone who loves me unconditionally. Scott has never felt the need to make excuses for my behavior. Why should he? I have a brain injury. Would someone make excuses for a spouse who has cancer, or MS, or any number of other medical conditions?

A friend, who is a caregiver, shared with me that she made a conscious decision early in her husband's brain injury to never make excuses for his behavior. If he acted out of bounds by conventional standards – then so be it. He was doing the best that he could and she refused to undermine his progress in social settings by making excuses for an occasional misstep. That does not mean that she did not work to help him relearn behavioral cues he had lost. But if his raw truthfulness was not the accepted etiquette of the group, she didn't worry about it.

Her message was loud and clear. She had made her decision when she married him many years ago. She was determined to always stand in his corner. Their love and understanding of traumatic brain injury humbles me. Both she and her husband are true champions in advocating for TBI survivors.

Although Scott never once said it – he made his decision over thirty years ago. He makes no excuses. He stands firmly in my corner.

It is wise to direct your anger towards problems – not people; to focus your energy on answers not excuses.
~ William Arthur Ward

The Secret Garden

There is a lovely, peaceful, green space at Shepherd called The Secret Garden. It is not a real secret because there is a sign mounted from the ceiling with an arrow pointing through the game room. Many patients and their family members go there for solitude, or perhaps to escape the hospital environment. I don't know how this space affects others, but it seems almost sacred to me. When I am in the Secret Garden, I speak in a subdued tone, and I relish the peacefulness.

It is filled with trees and art. It has a koi pond. In the spring and summer there are lovely flowers, many in raised beds so that wheelchair bound patients can help tend them. The flowers attract birds and butterflies to this mecca in the middle of the bustle of Atlanta. In mid-December there were no flowers, but it was still lovely.

I remember spending a Saturday afternoon in there with Scott. He had come to my room and had announced that he was taking me somewhere that I would really like. He wheeled me to the elevator, down endless corridors, and finally out into the secret garden. It was an especially mild December day. He gave me a weight shift, positioning my chair on the two back wheels, allowing the fractures still healing in my pelvis, tailbone, and two vertebrae in my spine to feel the blessed relief of not bearing my upper body weight.

He leaned my chair back so far that I imagined that I lay on cool green grass looking up through the trees at the clouds slowly drifting by overhead. I felt the sun and wind on my face and body, and pretended that I was home, on the grass beside Scott enjoying a beautiful day together. He was quiet and allowed me this time to daydream. It was marvelous.

Today, I still make the pilgrimage to the Secret Garden when I visit Shepherd as a peer visitor. I am flooded with so many memories. It was here that I began to accept that I would be forever changed. On my most recent peer visit I walked down the three steps from the door and remembered that not so long ago I was wheeled down the ramp. I sat on a bench close by the door and looked around. I felt again that I was in a sacred place. After a few moments of solitude in this wondrous space, I began to observe other patients and family members in various locations around the garden.

I looked over to the very spot where Scott had once held my chair and had allowed me to daydream of being anywhere but here, in this hospital. There, in our spot, sat a man. He had sustained a spinal cord injury and was in a wheelchair that mechanically altered the chair into a weight shift position, so that he, like me three years ago, reclined almost horizontal to the ground looking up through those same trees watching the clouds drift by. His wife sat on a nearby bench reading a book. He, like me, was alone in his thoughts. I prayed that he would find both the escape and the beginnings of acceptance that I discovered in the same spot not so long ago.

Maybe this is why the Secret Garden feels so sacred. For those who seek it, there is a spiritual communion and awakening, offering the seeker the beginning of acceptance and peace.

May your roots go down deep into the soil of God's marvelous love; and may you be able to feel and understand...how long, how wide, how deep, and how high his love really is; and to experience this love for yourselves, though it is so great that you will never see the end of it or fully know or understand it. And so at last you will be filled up with God himself.
Ephesians 3:17-19
~ NIV version as adapted by Debbie Kingston

Why Me?

'I used to think if only I had been delayed for just a few seconds longer I would not have had the car wreck, and my life would have been so much better. Then, one day, I realized that my life would not have been better, only the same. I would have continued to get up every day and I would still be plodding down the same path. Although I might have been physically healthier, does that necessarily mean better? I know perfectly healthy people who are miserable.

Life is made up of ordinary and extraordinary moments, and only God is worthy to measure the difference. What seems ordinary to us can be extraordinary in hindsight. People, who didn't realize they were making an impression on me, have immeasurably influenced me. They have changed the course of my life. Likewise, I have influenced others in ways I can't comprehend. The smallest act of kindness can have spiritual ramifications we never consider. When we give to others, we create waves of change in the spiritual light present in the world. Our thoughts, our words, our actions can create an extraordinary moment for others and change the course of a life.

I met my husband by walking into a local teen club when he was shooting a game of pool. Thirty minutes sooner or later and we would have missed each other. I can think of hundreds of examples in my life that were set in motion by being in the right place at the right time. Who understands the intent of God? Can we presume to think that only the events we agree with are the ones that God should allow? Can we honestly say that we would be better people if we experienced no pain, no loss, no regret in our lives? Should we only expect success and never failure? Aren't the greatest life lessons those that cost us the most? If every event were pleasant or easy, would we ever feel the exhilarating joy of achievement?

I begin to realize that there are no coincidences with God, no chance encounters, no unintended lessons in life. There is a plan and there are choices. God offers us great, and sometimes we settle for good, or even opt for bad, but ultimately the decision on what path to travel is ours.

Our lives, and the lives of our families, have been forever changed. Continually looking behind at the past is a time consuming mistake. Wishing for the past is much like staring into your rear view mirror. If you are concentrating on what's behind, how can you focus on what's ahead?

Life is so fleeting. We are here for such a short time; the blink of an eye, then our time is over. For me, the real question is no longer "Why did this happen to me, God?" I have come to understand that the most important questions to ask God do not begin with *why* – they begin with *how*. "*How* can I make the most of my time? *How* can I improve the quality of my life? *How* can I improve the lives of others? *How* can I determine your plan for me, God?"

Ask these questions of God, and watch the awe-inspiring power that created and plotted the universe set the course for your life.

"Trust in the Lord with all thine heart; and lean not unto thine own understanding. In all of thy ways acknowledge him, and he shall direct thy paths"
~ Proverbs 3:5-6

Know this First

Why did this happen to ME?

Know this first – God did not cause your catastrophe!

Some people get mad at God. They are overwhelmed by the pain and loss they face and blame their dilemma on God. They refuse to talk with him or to ask for his help just when they need him most. God is the power source! If we blame him for our current dilemma, we are cutting ourselves off from the help we need.

If you cut through your lamp's power cord, how would you light when it gets dark? It is that way with God. How can we find the energy, the faith, and the light we need to lead us out of darkness to heal effectively, if we have cut ourselves off from his power? I spent one year of my life in hospitals and in outpatient rehabilitation. I spent another three and half years having more surgeries than I can count and additional therapies. In that four and a half years, I observed that people who progress the slowest, suffer the most, and seem in the most pain and fear have asked the question, "Why me?" and have not worked out a satisfactory answer in their own heart. They are angry or bitter.

In the midst of catastrophe, it is inevitable to ask, "Why me?" I have come to believe that how this question is answered sets the foundation for healing.

Eight weeks after my accident, I had been at Shepherd for two weeks. It was late at night and the room was dark. Down the hall I heard someone moaning. I lay awake and in great pain, and thought, "Why did this happen to me?" As I thought about this, my personal answer allowed me to get past this *one greatest stumbling block*, so I could concentrate on healing.

I took a mental survey of my life. I was fifty years old. I had been married to a wonderful man for twenty-eight years. I had three healthy kids, a nice home, an interesting job, and many friends. I could remember perfect days when the weather had been lovely and I had felt on top of the world. And never once, in any of these miraculous moments, did I ever stop and ask God, "*Why m*e? What have I done to deserve such great blessings in my life?" Yet, now, when the rain had fallen into my life, the first thing I wanted to do was ask God, "Why me?" As I thought of it this way, I began to feel like a hypocrite.

Some believe, "If there really is a God, he would have prevented my accident or any illness." Some believe that there are no such things as accidents. They say that if I had listened to God sooner when he tried to get my attention, I would not have had my accident. In other words, if you don't listen to God when he whispers, then his next attempt to get your attention may cause you great pain or catastrophe.

"This then is the message which we have heard of him, God is light and in him is no darkness at all." 1 John 1:5 There is no darkness in God at all. None. Not one speck. What I experienced was definitely dark. Therefore it did not come from God. I have grown to see that God has set up universal laws that rule the universe. I cannot see gravity, but I know the principle, I know it exists. I cannot see faith, but I know the principle, and I know it exists. For every action there is a reaction; for every decision there is a consequence. God set our world in order; he made it the same for everyone. These universal laws apply to all of us. Having a relationship with God does not ensure that there won't be rain in our lives, but it does ensure that when it's storming God will be our umbrella.

There is darkness in the world, too. Sometimes good people must take an unexpected and unwanted journey through this darkness. Can anyone fully understand why this is necessary? I can say that the times of my greatest adversity have also been the times of my greatest spiritual growth.

Traumatic brain injury, spinal cord injury, MS, cancer, being a victim of violence, the death of a loved one – these all make for dark times. They do not come from the God of light and love. At times like this all of us will ask this question, "Why ME?" No one else can answer this question for you.

I can only share my truth as I understand it, and say that I have been there. I am absolutely convinced that until you can successfully answer this question to your own satisfaction, and eliminate bitterness from your heart and mind, your progress out of this darkness will be slower and harder to bear.

"For light I go directly to the Source of light, not to any of the reflections. Also I make it possible for more light to come to me by living up to the highest light I have. You cannot mistake light coming from the Source, for it comes with complete understanding so that you can explain it and discuss it."
~ Peace Pilgrim

The Comforter

After my accident Scott went to our local bank to discuss our finances, to determine what needed to be done to ensure our bills were paid even though he would be out of town much of the time. A week later, he returned home to a phone call from our local branch manager, asking if he could drop something off at the house. He brought a lovely, velvet comforter in jewel-tone colors.

He told Scott that his church had prayer over the comforter and he wanted me to use it while in the hospital. He believed it would bless me and aid me in healing. It was the perfect size to cover the top of a hospital bed, yet it didn't get in the way of the tubes, and other medical necessities. It was a beautiful gift. I never felt a chill lying under this wonderful comforter for five months. Today, it hangs in a prominent place on the wall to help me remember that when I needed it most, God sent me a comforter.

That name is perfect. It speaks to caring with love, personifying this covering. A subtle reminder of the spiritual comforter God has also given. "Comforter" is the word that Jesus Christ used to describe the Holy Spirit. It is the Holy Spirit that speaks truth to us. It is this quiet voice that each of us individually hears that guides us in our daily lives. It is this still, small voice, disguised as a thought, which encourages us and ultimately leads to peace.

"But the comforter, which is the Holy Spirit, whom the Father will send in my name, he shall teach you all things and bring all things to your remembrance, whatsoever I have said unto you. Peace I leave with you, my peace I give unto you; Not as the world giveth, give I unto you. Let not your heart be troubled neither let it be afraid." John 14: 26-27

This sustained me in my darkest trials. This enabled me to see beyond myself and to reach out to others in prayer, even when I was most fragile. This is what caused me to overcome obstacle after obstacle to achieve an independent life. It is this communion with God through the Comforter, the Holy Spirit, that has made all things possible for me.

But when the Comforter is come, whom I will send unto you from the Father, even the Spirit of truth, which proceedeth from the Father, he shall testify of me.
~John 16:26

Extraordinary Care

I first remember her as a blurred face leaning over me as I was wheeled out of Memorial University Medical Center for my transfer to Shepherd. She leaned over my stretcher and said, "If there is anything you need, please let me know." I don't think I responded. I just remember seeing her face and wondering, who was she? Then I saw her face again at Shepherd during lunch. She sat down beside me and spoke with me. I don't remember what she said. I just remember asking myself, "Who is this woman?" Did I know her?

Her name was Irma. After all of these years I still can't remember her official title. She is the trained medical professional assigned to work with me. It was months before I understood that Irma worked behind the scenes to help Scott acquire whatever resources I needed to begin to heal. It was a year before I realized that I could never handle all of the appointments, surgeries, forms, approvals, etc. on my own. Irma gave me the luxury of concentrating only on healing, because she expertly and quietly handled everything else. For seven years she has helped me in so many ways, that I am at a loss to list them all. I used to think of her as my advocate, but now I think of her as a trusted and cherished friend.

As a breast cancer survivor, she understood many of the challenges I faced. When my hair fell out she was a gentle listening ear. She is tough, fair, and has always been there for me. Like a velvet and steel glove, she intuitively knew when to listen compassionately and when to speak the hard but firm truths that kept me grounded and focused on healing. She knows more of the details of my medical procedures than anyone, including me. When I was released to go home, Irma worked with Scott to make remodeling decisions based on accommodations for my wheelchair. She even helped pick out the ceramic tile for my handicap accessible bathroom. She found reliable home care for me, visited me, and was available to me for whatever I needed. Irma has been my rock. She has blessed me in innumerable ways, but one great blessing was when she introduced me to Ivan.

Ivan has been my driver for seven years. He has taken me to and from more outpatient surgeries and therapies than I care to remember. He has loaded and unloaded my wheelchair, then my walker, and has witnessed my journey in healing closer than anyone but my family. He has been a constant reliable companion and a listening ear to all of my moods and challenges. I am one of his long-term clients and I hope that he considers me a friend too. In the early days I slept on the way home from my outpatient therapy. The entire day of therapy took all of my energy. So, for the one-hour trip home each afternoon he listened to me snore.

At this time my visits are more on the lines of a weekly transport and we argue politics, discuss family, and keep up with each other's lives. In all of this time he has never kept me waiting. Early in my therapy I was temporarily assigned a different driver and he left me waiting for hours. He had a car and the one-hour commute into Atlanta and back was a painful ordeal. Ivan has a van and the seat is almost as comfortable as a reclining chair. Most important is that his driving is not erratic. He is probably the best driver I know. I hesitate to admit this because if Ivan reads this he will never let me forget it. Riding with Ivan has been easy, because he genuinely cares for others and his care of me has been exceptional.

If not for the wreck, I would have missed out on meeting these two wonderful people and my life would have been poorer. There are so many doctors, nurses, and therapists, etc. who impact your life when you are on a long-term journey to health. They all play an important part, but those who provide a daily service not considered life altering are paramount in the healing process. Within turbulence there can be peace.

Meeting Irma and Ivan has been the great peaceful reminder that this too shall pass. The extraordinary care that they have given me over the course of seven years is directly responsible for my positive improvements, and regaining my independence. They provided a multitude of little blessings that lifted me in small but steady ways culminating in better health and a renewed and positive sense of self. Can there be a better definition of love?

Too often we underestimate the power of a touch, a smile, a kind word, a listening ear, an honest compliment, or the smallest act of caring, all of which have the potential to turn a life around. ~ Leo Biscaglia

Acceptance

It happened quietly and without fanfare. There was no shining moment that was indelibly marked when I accepted the changes in myself caused by my brain injury. Acceptance came slowly, the breathing in of everyday life, like the change of the seasons. The hot, humid days of summer were sprinkled with days of tangy autumn breezes. Then, one day I noticed that the trees were ablaze in crimson, gold, burgundy, and orange. Acceptance, like autumn, had finally arrived.

The injured brain struggles to fit the old preferences into a new paradigm of self that no longer works. It takes time to determine what pieces fit and what pieces should be discarded. This puzzle once had all of the correct pieces packaged neatly in the box. Without acceptance there is the frustration of continually cramming an old piece that will not fit into an opening of a new puzzle. Yearning for the old life is an exasperating waste of time. I realize that I have spent years trying to shove the wrong pieces into this puzzle in so many places. I don't have the luxury of throwing away this damaged box. This is the only brain I have. I must find the correct pieces to rebuild a new picture of my life that is both satisfying and functional for me.

Acceptance was a natural timing, like a change in season, which finally allowed me to begin to select the proper pieces to rebuild my life. I am the product of all that I have experienced, all that I have dreamed, all that I know, all that I can remember. The intricacies of this personal puzzle are found in my story and the history of my life. These foundational pieces still fit the puzzle.

The challenge of living with my traumatic brain injury is to understand that I possess puzzle pieces that, in many ways, became instantly obsolete. I felt imprisoned in a puzzle where many pieces no longer fit. Preferences in what I like to eat, to wear, what music soothes me, what art inspires me, what I like to do for pleasure – all of this has changed.

It has taken more than four years for me to comprehend this truth, and to learn and accept these changes. I must seek new pieces that fit who I am today. It is an ongoing process that can be overwhelming and frustrating one day, and satisfying and illuminating in the next. It is a tough puzzle that must be reworked piece by piece to achieve independent living. Honestly understanding which pieces must be reinforced with notepads, sticky notes, calendars, and lists to fit properly takes time and patience.

Acceptance has led me to finally bury those old pieces. Every moment of independent achievement in the new self becomes another shovel of dirt that buries the old self. Time officiates this process in a silent unspoken sermon. The physical and mental part of me that was catastrophically changed in an instant becomes the foundation that I build on. I begin to understand that I was a mere shadow when compared to the woman who stands today. It is a great paradox.

This mind, that has suffered traumatic injury, has spent years yearning for the former self, not understanding that the most important part of me not only survived, but has also thrived. The core of who I am is the spiritual self that has broken free from the confines of the former life. It is ongoing, it is ever changing, and it can be simultaneously exhilarating and terrifying. It is life, as I know it now.

It is the new me.

Of course there is no formula for success
except perhaps an unconditional acceptance
of life and what it brings.
~ Arthur Rubenstein

The New Us

I look out of my window and I see the autumn breeze ripple the water across our lake. I consider how one disturbance in one part of the lake causes a disturbance across the whole lake.

As my husband Scott told me not long after my injury, "You know Diane, your accident didn't just happen to you. It happened to all of us." That is both the tragedy and the glory of surviving a traumatic brain injury.

I remember clearly when my daughter Kelly and I decided to swim in the lake. I used to love to swim, but had not been able, due to my colostomy. This was the first summer since my reversal surgery. We both put on our swimsuits and walked to the dock. She jumped into the water with wild abandon and came up laughing. I felt myself rooted to the dock in some inexplicable fear.

She yelled, "Come on in Mom. The water feels great." And still I could not move. She swam closer to the dock. "Are you all right?" she asked.

I heard myself answer, "I'm scared," and realized that I sounded like I had in second grade when my Dad had taught me to swim.

She scrutinized me carefully, and then she began to clap her hands and say, "Come on, Momma. You can do it. Just close your eyes and jump. I'm right here.

You'll be fine. Trust me, I won't let anything bad happen."

I gave a nervous laugh. *Wasn't this what I had said to her when she was learning to swim?* Under her watchful eyes and with great encouragement, I finally summoned the courage to jump. The water felt glorious and as an added bonus our new puppy jumped in, too. All three of us swam. I could no longer swim in the ways I used to, but I was a fierce dog paddler. So the puppy and I dog paddled to our hearts' content as Kelly swam around us calling out encouragement to us both.

That afternoon is etched into my heart. My teenaged daughter had easily swapped roles and had become the adult when I required it. It felt wonderful to be accepted for exactly who I was while I stood so fearful on that dock. My new perception of myself is sometimes shaky, but my family's acceptance of the new us is rock solid. I can be open about my thoughts and my family will accept it as 'my' truth.

In the final Harry Potter novel, *Harry Potter and the Deathly Hallows*, a conversation between Harry and Dumbledore concludes with Harry asking Dumbledore, "Is this real? Or has this been happening inside my head?"

Dumbledore replies, "Of course it is happening inside your head, Harry, but why on earth should that mean that it is not real?"

Anxiety, lack of self-confidence, inexplicable fears that sometimes overwhelm me emotionally, may not have a rational reason, but they are real – at least to me. Added to these feelings is a diminished short-term memory, lack of concentration and inability to function well in stressful situations. Having people around who love you, who will accept these moments and become what you need to overcome them, is a precious gift.

The role of the caregiver is essential in the life of a traumatic brain injury survivor because as Scott said, "It happened to all of us." We have all been forever changed and the traditional roles of parent and child, or spouse do not always apply. Sometimes the chameleon like ability to become what the other person needs is the only answer. It takes courage, honesty, and love for others in the family for everyone to regain their own security and comfort level in this new family unit. It is not easy to find the fluidity to function in family roles that are out of character, but maintaining a sense of humor can lighten the darker moments of accepting this changing family dynamic.

It takes time to become the new us.

The possibility of stepping into a higher plane is quite real for everyone. It requires no force or effort or sacrifice. It involves little more than changing our ideas about what is normal. ~ Deepak Chopra

The Last Word

My room was located on the back hall of the ABI unit when I was a patient. I have walked past it twice since I was released, and each time I choke with emotion as the memories flood my mind. That room is where I spent throbbing pain-filled nights that seemed to have no end. It is where I faced my fear alone in the dark. It is where I first began to realize that my life had been changed forever. If I arrive early to volunteer at Shepherd, I avoid this hall and visit the Secret Garden instead.

On a recent visit I walked the path within the Secret Garden and noticed large rocks mixed among the raised beds of flowers. These rocks were approximately eight to twelve inches tall. Patients from the ABI and SCI units had painted all of them. Knowing that people in the early stages of treatment from traumatic brain or spinal cord injury had painted these rocks made them all the more fascinating.

Many bore emblems and colors of college football teams. Others were painted in bright colors had quotes on them. Someone had painted a lovely red rose on one with the words, "I am very thankful" beneath the rose. I paused to consider this stone. So many people don't feel thankful and they walk on two legs at their leisure. They remember and think without any prompts at all. I used to be one of them. Now I share the rose stone author's view and I am very thankful, too. Another rock bore the statement, "God is my great physician."

As I thought about this, the paint therapy teacher approached. She pointed out a rock that had been painted by a quadriplegic. Unable to use his hands he had held the paintbrush in his mouth and daubed paint onto the stone in a variety of vibrant colors. She told me that the last color he had painted was yellow. I noticed the round blob of yellow paint located exactly in the center of the stone. He had asked her to paint a smiley face in it.

This rock was most special to her because it took the most effort to paint. After she walked away, I stood for many minutes staring at it. I began to understand that the smiley face was the artist's credo, a declaration of independence from a body that no longer worked. He still had his mind. He realized that he could still control what he thought. The smiley face represented his decision of how he chose to face his new life.

Thinking of these rocks as the personal credo of the patients who had painted each, I studied them more closely. Several quoted scriptures. "I can do all things through Christ which strengtheneth me" was on one and it included a drawing of a flexed arm muscle and even included a copy of the painter's tattoo on his arm. Another rock pictured a rainbow and a dove, symbols of promise and peace. They demonstrated the heart of one who had attained a feeling of calm despite the great turbulence of tragedy.

Finally, I spied a rock that spoke loudest to me. It had been painted entirely in bright orange. Dark blue, hand painted, letters in a shaky handwriting that had run in several places, proclaimed, "The last word isn't written." I considered the person who had taken the time to send this message out as a great call for hope. It was the silent answer to every negative statement directed toward someone in the battle of his or her life to regain health. You may never walk again – *the last word isn't written*. You may never think clearly again – *the last word isn't written*. You may never speak again – *the last word isn't written*.

Who will write my last word? Only I can do that. Only I can write the message for each day of my life. I awake each morning to a blank rock. Only I control what will be painted onto my rock for that day. Will my brushstroke write faith or fear, love or apathy, acceptance or bitterness? I am the author of my rock. No one else can write my future. Doctors, family, friends, may tell me what they think is in store for me, but *the last word isn't written*. They cannot paint on my rock. Only my faith and actions press the paintbrush to stone. As the other rock had proclaimed loud and clear, "God is my great physician."

When I left the Secret Garden, I went back to the ABI unit to prepare for the Peer Visitor meeting. Before going into the conference room, I walked by my old room. I stood in the empty hall and looked into an empty room. I felt painful memories rush toward me. Silently I spoke to the room. "You are my past and I will leave you here. I will learn from you, but I will not let you hurt me anymore. I have more important things to do today, because the last word isn't written." I turned my back to the room and walked away.

We are what we think. All that we are arises with our thoughts. With our thoughts, we make the world.
~ Buddha

Acknowledgements

This book has been a seven-year project. In those years, so many people have helped and encouraged me that I may forget to thank someone. Should this happen, I ask your pardon and hope you will know that your help is much appreciated.

Thank you to:

- My friends and mentors in the Carrollton Creative Writers Club (CCWC) who have been invaluable with knowledge and advice on every phase of writing and publishing a book. Your critiques of my stories have made this book something I can be proud of.
- Tom Cook, Amber Pickle and Donna Spivey, who read and edited this at the end, and gave me the truth.
- Zan Marie Steadham, my editor, and fellow scribe, whose encouragement and dedication in the final edit of this book, was a great blessing.
- John Bell at Vabella Publishing for making this process so easy.
- Jesse Duke for his perfect cover art for the front of the book.

- Brady Parks for designing the front and back cover of the book, and so much more.
- Scott, Anthony, Kelly, Kacy, Doug, Denise, Brandon, Mom, Diane, Kendra Moon, Linda Young, Dr. Damond Logsdon, Patsy White Smith, Renee Conner, and anyone else who read parts, or the entire book in the early stages and offered encouragement.

Thank you to those who stood by me during my recovery. Thank you:

- Diane Reeves, you were my greatest champion and friend in deed, and for all family and friends who came to visit – thank you for your love.
- Ralph Riley for the well-timed flowers recorded in God's Timetable.
- Friends and former colleagues at The National Association of Women in Construction (NAWIC), BE&K Inc., and Atlanta Technical College, whose prayers, cards, phone calls, and love sustained me.
- Kim Patterson for your help.
- Clay Hicks, and David Byrd, for keeping vigil, and acting as family, until my family arrived.
- The people in my community of Carrollton, Georgia, who prayed for me and helped my husband and children, handle this tragedy.
- Every person who came to visit. I cannot name you all, but your visits helped me hang on.

Thank you to the medical professionals in Savannah and Atlanta, who gave me their best effort, culminating in my ability to lead a useful and fulfilling life. Special thanks go to:

- The staff at Memorial University Hospital, the Shepherd family, and the staff at Shepherd and Pathways.
- My case manager Kendra Moon for her help while at Pathways, and on this book.
- Dr. Gerald Bilsky, my doctor for over seven years for your skill and friendship.
- Irma and Ivan Bloch for years of caring and support.
- Tommy Owens, DDS, for giving me back my smile and for inspiring me to raise money for TBI.
- Dr. Errol Bailey, for your skill and dedication to your profession. You performed a miracle on my feet and when I walk without pain, I have you to thank.
- Every surgeon who has worked on me. I cannot remember all of you by name, and I was asleep while you worked, but my eyes are wide open now and I am thankful for your skill.
- Dr. Damond Logsdon, PhD, my psychologist, who understands brain injury better than anyone other than a TBI survivor, and has helped me regain my life.

Thank you to my attorneys, Bill Stemberger (general law), Susan Sadow (workers compensation), Pam Atkinson (social security), and Jeff Warnike (disability insurance), for your help when most needed. I highly recommend you to anyone who finds himself/herself in my predicament.

Thanks and love to my parents, Margaret and Gordon Lane, who got out of bed in the middle of the night and came to Savannah, and have always, been there for me. Thanks go to my brother and sister-in-law, Doug and Denise, nephew, Brandon, and niece, Jackie, who were, and still are, there for me. Denise, your email prayer chain was only one of the many things you did for me. You and I both know that your email updates assembled a group of Prayer Warriors who remembered me in prayer, and this made all the difference.

Thank you Ethel Quimby, my mom-in-law, my friend, a great blessing in my life, and a frequent visitor when I needed her most. Thank you to my extended family – Aunt Bonnie, Uncle I O, Mike, Luke and Isabel Johnson, Aunt Billie Sue, Uncle Teddy, Danny, Andy, and Deborah, and Betty Riley – for your prayers, visits, and loving support.

And a thank you so great that it cannot be spoken in words, but must somehow be expressed to Scott who is the great gift of love that God has given me. Your love and commitment are my inspiration. Anthony, Kelly, and Kacy – this happened to us all and you are my heart! You four are the reason I fought so hard to survive, and continue to fight for my health. Your unconditional love and support have carried me far beyond what I ever dreamed I could accomplish. I Love You.

All praise to God for his grace, and great blessings to my family and to me.

Diane Quimby is a former educator, corporate training manager, and journeyman carpenter. She taught carpentry at Atlanta Technical College and was the 1998 recipient of the Rick Perkins Award, Teacher of the Year for post-secondary teachers in Georgia. She was the first woman in Atlanta local #3024 to achieve journeyman status, and the first woman department chair of a skilled trades division in a technical college in Georgia.

While working at BE&K Construction Inc. as manager of training, she designed and directed an annual free one-week Girls Construction Summer Camp. After recovering from her car accident she co-founded Mentoring A Girl in Construction (MAGIC) Summer Camp that reaches high school girls across the nation.

Diane serves on the Georgia Brain & Spinal Injury Trust Fund Commission (BSITF) Advisory Committee, and is a volunteer in the Traumatic Brain Injury Peer Visiting Program at the Shepherd Center. She has a BS in Education and an MA in Adult Education.

As a public speaker, she shares her story at conferences and seminars offering hope to traumatic brain injury survivors and caregivers. She shares her unique experiences and lessons learned on her continuing journey of healing in her book, *Head Lights for Dark Roads: Packing Humor and Hope for the Unexpected Trip through Traumatic Brain Injury*. All profits from the sale of her book are donated to TBI organizations. You can contact Diane at her blog: www.tbi-411.blogspot.com
Or her email address: dianequimbytbi@gmail.com.